Everything You Always

Wanted To Know About

Energy

But Were Too Tired To Ask

by Dr. Paul Varnas & Barbara J. Stepp, CH

Library of Congress
Cataloging-in-Publication Data
Varnas, Paul G.
Stepp, Barbara J.
Everything you always wanted to know
about energy, but were too tired to ask
by Paul G. Varnas & Barbara J. Stepp
©1996 Paul G. Varnas & Barbara J. Stepp
ISBN 0-9649818-0-7

Trademark acknowledgments: ADP², Advil², Aleve², Armor-All², Birkenstock², Biotics², Chee-tos², Coke², Congaplex™, Di-Gel², Diet Coke², Equal², Hershey's², Holsum², Max-EPA², Natural Ovens of Manitowoc, WI, Neuro Linguistic Programming, Nutrasweet², Nystatin², Optifast², Prozac², Rolex², Smucker's², Styrofoam², Technicolor², Twix², Tylenol², Vita-Mix², Zinc Tally².

I'd like to dedicate my work here to my three
sources of fatigue, Alanna, Adam and Catherine.

Dr. Paul G.Varnas

...And to my three sources of energy,
Richard Bandler, Tony Robbins and God.
(but not necessarily in that order)

Barbara J. Stepp, CH

table of contents

v

table of contents

foreword

This program resulted from a team effort between Barbara Stepp and myself. I had finished the first rough draft of the manuscript when I began to take Barbara's class in Neuro Linguistic Programming. Her class opened up for me many possibilities, both for my practice and for what this book could potentially be.

Neuro Linguistic Programming is so amazing and so effective that I became very excited about what the benefits could be to my patients, my students and my readers. I asked Barbara to write the exercises and create the tape set that turned this from a pretty good health book into a complete system that can virtually guarantee you more energy than you ever thought possible.

In the biblical story of creation, God took dust and formed man. He then breathed into the dust and gave the man life and a soul. Barbara's contribution to this package is like that breath of life.

A good model for health is an equilateral triangle. The three sides of the triangle are the components necessary for good health. They are chemical balance, structural balance and mental (or spiritual) balance. Before the addition of Barbara's exercises and tapes, this book was lacking information about the mental side of the triangle.

The exercises and information about Neuro Linguistic Programming are vital to this program's effectiveness. After all, the mind can heal the body. It is a powerful tool that will provide you with virtually anything you ask of it. Doctors are discovering more and more the importance of attitude and state of mind in healing.

Since the manuscript was just about finished when Barbara and I met, we decided not to completely rewrite it, but to improve it. Since I had written the book conversationally, in the first person, we left it that way. Barbara's contributions are all through the text, but the style of the book is from my point of view. It leaves the impression that the book is entirely mine. That isn't the case. I merely provided the dust for Barbara's breath of life.

Paul G. Varnas

foreword

Throughout my life I have had many challenges to my health. Some of my experiences qualify as real medical nightmares. I made great progress and improvement with my health through NLP, hypnosis and the power of the mind. Through the power of my brain and through the types of techniques that you will learn in this package I moved from being a semi-invalid to being a scuba diver, sky diver and rock climber. I enjoy a very active lifestyle, full of adventure.

Through all this, however, my health was still not perfect. I experienced extreme physical pain on a regular basis. My training enabled me to tune out the pain and maintain my active lifestyle, but I had to take time and energy to focus on feeling good.

There is quite a difference between overcoming pain and being pain-free. I had to work very hard in order to not experience the pain and the signals my nervous system was giving to me.

As a doctor and friend, Paul helped me to learn to listen to my body. He made me realize that I should listen to my body's messages, rather than to just focus on overcoming them with my mind. His model of health is that of an equilateral triangle consiting of mind (or spirit), biochemical, and structural. All areas of health need attention. I had put all of my eggs in one basket, the mental, and was having a hard time.

Working with him was a major revelation to me as I realized the connection, the interdependence between the mind and the body. By taking care of my physical health, I was able to free myself from pain and not spend so much time and energy to make my nervous system stop reminding me of my physical problems.

The result of our mutual revelations is this book and tape program. Enjoy!

Barbara J. Stepp

preface

This book is part of a set that includes six audiotapes and a workbook. The tape set is entitled "30 Days to Total Energy". It contains hypnosis and Neuro Linguistic Programming exercises to make following the advice in this book easy. The tapes have information, exercises and hypnotic inductions that are designed to accompany this book and facilitate your return to health and energy.

Both this book and the tape set are designed to stand on their own. The tapes contain a brief outline of the health advice contained in this book. This book contains written exercises similar to those contained in the tape set. Each component of the package, however, compliments the other.

The topics covered on the tapes are as follows.

① **Habits.** Getting rid of undesired habits. Developing desired habits.

② **Stress.** NLP exercises and self-hypnosis to eliminate stress.

③ **Sleep.** Getting to sleep, staying asleep and waking feeling rested.

④ **Managing your state of mind/Controlling your Emotions.** Creating energy at a moment's notice.

⑤ **Healing and psychoneuroimmunology.** Exercise to help the mind heal the body.

⑥ **Creating a compelling future.** Using your time line to create what you want in life.

Each of the above topics is covered in the book. The tapes, however, go into greater detail and also take you through the exercises, step by step. To order the tapes, call 800-672-2250.

acknowledgments

We would like to acknowledge Marti Marsden and Chi Stoker at Jackson Gray, Inc. for their wonderful work in the design of this book. We have a new appreciation of the hard work and creativity that goes into the stages of producing a book. We will never look at a book cover the same way again.

We would like to also acknowledge Jane Crouse for her fine work in editing this manuscript and making our words understandable. Also, Jane should be thanked for her indulgence in allowing us to completely ignore her advice for Part 3 of this book.

Ralph Valatka should also be recognized for his production work and for making the tape set possible.

Also, a special thank you to Karen Thorne for being the rudder of our ship and for making all of this work.

introduction

One of my nightmares is one where I receive a letter from the law offices of McGreedy, Larsen and Snatch. The letter states that their client, a Mr. I.M. Needlebrain read one of my books and pursued a course of self-treatment. It goes on to tell me that the unfortunate Mr. Needlebrain had been suffering from a case of Fecalith Systematica, and had he sought out proper medical assistance, he could have been easily cured with a course of antibiotics and an enema.

The letter goes on to say that reading the book convinced Mr. Needlebrain that he could treat himself. The fact that the book did not advise him of the possibility that he had Fecalith Systematica constitutes negligence. As a result, he wasted valuable time trying questionable treatments, while his health continued to decline. His health became worse, and he finally went into a coma and is not expected to live. His estranged family, overcome with grief, is suing for $50 million, my Mad magazine collection and my firstborn child.

The point is, don't try to be your own doctor. I don't have $50 million dollars, my mother burned my Mad magazine collection in 1976 and my firstborn is quite a handful. (Besides she'd be about 43 by the time all of the court proceedings were over.)

Fatigue is a symptom that is present in many serious diseases including cancer, diabetes and AIDS. No book, not even one as brilliantly written as this one, can anticipate every possible health problem or be a substitute for proper health care.

So why write a book? Why not just have a single sentence: "See your doctor." There are two reasons. First, and most importantly, it's hard to get people to shell out their hard-earned dollars for a single sentence. Second, most people who suffer with fatigue don't get much help from their doctors. Medical doctors seldom pay attention to, or even believe in the types of problems that cause fatigue. Patients are often told that their problem is stress or depression. They may even be put on Prozac or some other mind-altering drug.

Even though it is important to rule out serious disease, most people who are fatigued don't have a serious disease. Most of you reading this book have been to the doctor, had serious disease ruled out and have not been given a solution.

The amount of energy you have is proportional to how healthy you are. Being healthy is not just a matter of not being sick. Health is when all of the body's organs and systems are functioning optimally. If the organs and systems of your body are not working at their best, you become fatigued.

Proper nutrition, activity, waste removal, rest and genetics are all vital to optimum health. If these components are not supplied, the body begins a progression that ends in disease.

Poor nutrition, inactivity, improper waste removal and lack of rest, do not immediately cause health problems. When denied the necessary components of health, however, individual cells begin to function poorly. Health is less than optimal, but there are no symptoms, at least at first.

When I was in my twenties I did a pretty good job of making sure my cells didn't function optimally. At age 21, Thomas Edison had his first invention. At age 21, I was concerned about who shot J.R. and whether or not the Detroit Tigers would win the pennant. Stanley Wriniarski and I would see which one of us could consume the most depth charges. I would say things like, "I'll feel better after I throw up." "Let's go on a road trip, I can catch up on my sleep on Wednesday." Or I could be heard saying to women, "Come on honey, let's do it again." (Actually, this part is fantasy. I was pretty obnoxious and wasn't given much opportunity for that sort of thing. The point is, I could have said this if I didn't have my personality to act as birth control.) I could also be heard to say, "I'll have extra cheese and sausage on that pizza."

People would say things to me like, "How do you eat so much crap and not gain weight?" I ate food from the three major food groups: starch, grease and sugar. My idea of eating vegetables was mushrooms and tomato sauce on a pizza. (In fact, after the Reagan administration declared that ketchup was a vegetable, I began to feel that I was a real health nut.)

That sort of thing works for a while, but in time the abuse takes its toll. Poor cellular function, over a period of time, leads to enzyme and hormonal systems that function suboptimally. Nothing is really wrong yet, but you don't feel as good as you once did. In my thirties, I gave up Jack Daniels for white wine. I started trying to get some exercise and began eating more chicken. I could stay out all night, if it was for something important, but then I'd really need to catch up on my sleep the next day. I said things like, "You guys go on ahead, I'm going to stay home tonight and get some rest." "Give me a diet Coke with that." To my girlfriend (my body was falling apart, but my personality had improved), I'd say things like "Honest honey, this kind of thing has *never* happened before."

People would say things to me like, "Looks like you've put on a couple of pounds," and "You look so tired. Are you sure you feel all right?"

After a while, symptoms begin to appear. Fatigue becomes a regular occurrence. In my forties I really began to look forward to sleeping in. I'd say things like, "You know, I tried that new Aleve, and I think I like it better than Advil." "I gave up running, it bothered my knees too much." "Honey, can we do it tomorrow night instead? I want to watch the 'Gilligan's Island Retrospective' tonight." "You know I take better care of myself than I ever used to, but I'm so tired all of the time."

Years of abuse can lead to other symptoms, like dry skin, digestive problems, PMS, headaches, joint pain and, of course, fatigue. Even with the presence of symptoms, there may not be a problem or a diagnosable disease that can be identified by a doctor. As health begins to decline, signs of disease begin to appear. Signs are things that show up in diagnostic and laboratory tests. Finally the doctor has a disease that he or she can name and treat. In most cases, however, by the time a disease can be found, health has been in decline long before the signs and symptoms of disease were present.

Poor health is usually the result of the following progression: Bad habits, lack of necessary components of health → poor cell function → poor enzyme function → poor endocrine function → poor immune system function → malaise → symptoms → signs, or diagnosable disease.

You never hear someone say, "Yesterday I came down with cancer." Chronic disease does not just happen all of a sudden. It evolves after a departure from ideal health.

Even infectious disease needs a relatively unhealthy body to find a home. The bubonic plague killed half of the people in Europe in the fourteenth century. That means the other half didn't get the disease; they were healthier.

We say things like, "Yesterday I caught a cold." That implies that everyone around you "missed" the cold. The germs, with Michael Jordan-like moves, faked right, spun left, avoiding everyone else and slam-dunked into you. At work, school or any place where a lot of people are together, there are people who are sick all of the time and there are people who are never sick. Do the germs keep missing the same people all of the time? Of course not. People who don't get sick have better cell function, enzyme function, hormone function, immune system function and better overall health.

Wouldn't it be wise to treat your health before you developed a disease? If your car runs reasonably well and you take it to a mechanic, he doesn't say, "There's nothing wrong with your car, bring it to me when it doesn't run." A car has need of a mechanic, even when it is running. It needs regular maintenance to keep it running. The mechanic will change the oil and spark plugs in an otherwise "healthy" car. He doesn't wait until the engine locks up from lack of oil.

Many members of the medical profession should take lessons from mechanics. Doctors often do a poor job of taking care of health. They need a disease to fight before they can be effective. They are a lot like my brother. Tony always drives a large American car, made in the previous decade. One day I was in his car and it was making a very strange noise. I asked him what it was and he said that he didn't know. I asked him if he was worried about what it might be. His reply was, "When it breaks down, I'll know what the noise was."

My brother could have been a doctor. When there's disease present, they know exactly what to do. If there is a slight aberration of normal physiology, or a vague symptom, they're at a loss. Modern medicine is sickness oriented and most people suffering from fatigue are not sick. They just aren't very healthy.

Fatigue is the most common symptom of poor health. A person who is fatigued usually has normal lab tests and no disease that can be diagnosed by a doctor. Just because a disease isn't present doesn't mean that fatigue can't be treated. Doing things that promote health, the equivalent of changing the oil and spark plugs in a car, will cure fatigue.

The way to have all of the energy that you want is to develop healthy habits. Isn't it wiser to begin to return to ideal health than it is to wait until you have a disease that your doctor can name and give you a drug or other medical treatment?

We live in a time of skyrocketing medical costs. When it is discussed on the news, it is always called "health care." Medical intervention after a lifetime of ignoring health is expensive, but it isn't health care; it's sickness care. Sickness care is expensive; health care is actually pretty inexpensive.

We tend to want to abuse our bodies for a lifetime, and when we start having problems, we want to go to a doctor and have it fixed (preferably without any inconvenience or pain). A lot of the health dollar is spent on new technology and extensive treatment for serious diseases. Very little is spent on prevention or education.

Many people come into the offices of health care practitioners complaining about fatigue, skin problems, sinusitis, digestive disorders and other chronic problems. Few see the connection between their lifestyle and how they feel.

Alice was an artist who not only suffered from fatigue, but also had a horrible skin rash on her hands. They cracked, bled and were very painful. She had been to an internist, an allergist and a dermatologist and was unable to get a satisfactory diagnosis or an effective treatment. Combined, her doctors had close to 30 years of education among them. She was being treated with a steroid ointment that didn't seem to do her much good.

When she came into my office she was told to write down all of the food she consumed for one week. A typical day's food for her was as follows: Eight cups of coffee, butterscotch pudding and a pork chop. And that was a good day. She ate only one meal per day. She ate no fruits or vegetables. She drank no water, only coffee.

I convinced her to change her diet. She was motivated because her hands had gotten so bad that she couldn't work. After a few weeks of proper eating and some vitamin supplementation, her rash was almost completely healed.

The cure was so simple that it was laughable that she had so much trouble getting help. She only needed someone to treat the patient who had the rash and not simply treat the rash.

How expensive was it for her to see an internist and two specialists, have tests and fill prescriptions? The cost of her sickness care was much

6

more than the cost of what returned her to health, a simple change in her diet. Doctors' visits, tests and drugs are much more expensive than water, vegetables and other healthy food. Sickness care is much more expensive than health care.

No one took the time to ask Alice what she was eating or how she lived. Her doctors looked at the rash, compared it to other rashes they had seen and gave her the drug that usually worked for rashes. The problem wasn't that her doctors weren't skilled or dedicated. The problem was one of philosophy. Thinking of an illness as an enemy to be destroyed is often not as effective as helping the body return to normal physiology. They were treating the disease and not the whole body.

Most patients suffering from fatigue are often guilty of the same kind of neglect as Alice. They don't recognize the connection between diet and lifestyle and how they feel.

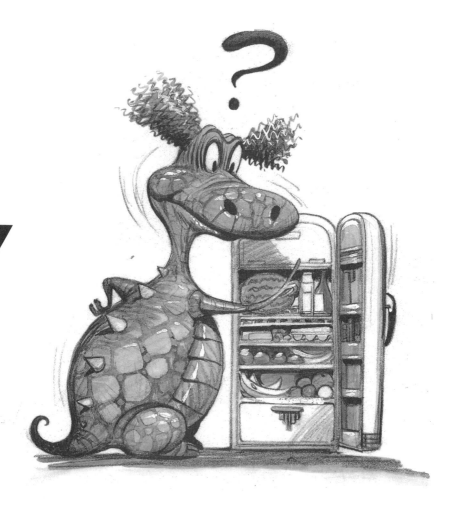

This part of the book contains information about general health and energy. Most people who are fatigued lack energy because their health habits are less than perfect. The information and advice contained in this part will benefit anyone, no matter what their health issues are, because the rules for staying healthy are the same for all of us.

How Your Habits Affect the Way You Feel

Simple changes in your day-to-day habits will give you more energy than you thought possible. Supplying your body with its basic needs will ensure good health. Being healthy means having plenty of energy.

If a car doesn't start or run well, the first thing you do is to make sure that it has gas and that the battery is charged. You put in new spark plugs or make sure that the fuel filter is clean. You don't immediately overhaul the engine. You check for small, common things that are easily repaired.

This is how you should approach your health. Just as a car needs gas, oil, electricity and occasional cleaning and replacement of components, the body needs oxygen, nutrients, proper elimination of waste, structural stability and movement. Unfortunately, most of us take better care of our cars than we do our bodies.

Your body is made up of billions of cells. Each cell is like a tiny factory that needs oxygen, nutrients and water and needs to eliminate waste in order to continue to function and produce its products. If your cells are healthy, you are healthy. If you are healthy, you have plenty of energy. Most people going on the 30-day program outlined at the end of this section will feel an incredible amount of energy. The beauty of it is that it doesn't matter what's wrong with you. If you are under the care of a doctor and are waiting for the results of tests, this part of the book can help you. If you are in the process of finding out if you have a disease or some kind of treatable pathology, this part of the book can still help you. There is nothing here that will interfere with any medical treatment.

Oxygen, Air, Breathing and Sinuses

The most important thing your body needs is oxygen. Denying your body oxygen will kill it faster than denying it anything else. You can live for weeks without food, for days without water, but only for minutes without oxygen. We all take breathing for granted, but it is the most important thing we do. **It defines life.**

Yoga and various martial arts recognize the importance of breathing. In yoga there are a variety of breathing exercises such as the cleansing breath or the breath of fire. In yoga, Pranayama is the rhythmic control of breath. According to the book, *Light on Pranayama* by B.K.S. Iyengar, during normal inhalation, an average person takes in about 500 cubic centimeters of air. During deep inhalation, the volume is six times as great. The Yogis believed that deep breathing energizes the body and cleanses the nadis, which are organs of the "subtle" body. In other words, there are not only physical and mental benefits to deep breathing, but also spiritual benefits.

Most of us breathe too shallowly and do not get good oxygenation of our tissues with each breath. Deep breathing can, at the same time, relax you and energize you. Try it now. Exhale and force all of the air out of your lungs. Slowly, deeply breathe the air back in. Use your diaphragm and fill your lungs to capacity. Pause for a few seconds with your lungs full. Exhale, even more slowly than you inhaled; take twice as long to exhale as you did to inhale. Force all of the air out of your lungs. Slowly inhale again and repeat the process. Do this for 10 breaths.

Notice the difference in how you feel after doing the deep breathing. If you didn't do the exercise, please do it now. It will make a difference in how you feel, and it will demonstrate to you just how much deep breathing can energize you. Deep breathing does two things. It delivers oxygen to the tissues and it increases lymphatic circulation.

Lymph is fluid that seeps from the capillaries and bathes all of the cells. The lymphatic system is sort of a storm sewer for the bloodstream and is also a key part of the immune system. It removes waste products from the cells like a storm sewer, gathering runoff from the bloodstream and wastes from the cells. It is also one of the major routes for absorption of nutrients from the digestive system. If lymphatic flow is sluggish, your body's cells sit in their own waste. The cells also do not receive sufficient oxygen or nutrients.

Deep breathing increases the flow of lymph. When you breathe deeply, you get oxygen to your cells and you help them to remove waste. The effects are felt almost immediately.

Sinuses

Another thing that interferes with your tissues getting enough oxygen is air pollution. The air is full of nitrogen and sulfur compounds, hydrocarbons and particulate waste. The poisons in the air decrease the efficiency of your lungs and present your body with a toxic burden.

Air pollution has created an explosion in the number of cases of sinusitis, which is the most common disease in America. There are over 34 million sufferers nationwide.

Sinuses are air pockets within the skull. It is believed that they exist to help control air pressure. Each sinus is connected to the nasal passage by a narrow canal called an ostium. The canals are about the width of a pencil lead. Each ostium is lined with a mucous membrane, which is tissue similar to the lining of the inside of the nose and mouth. The ostea are the connections between the sinuses and the outside.

Air pollution, allergies and smoking can irritate the ostea and cause the mucous membranes lining the canals to swell, closing the ostea. When the ostea are closed, pressure cannot be released from the sinus, creating a stuffy feeling and even sinus headaches.

Sinus infections become common because the sinuses frequently become full of mucous and become a breeding ground for bacteria. Often sufferers don't even know they have a sinus infection. They believe that it is a cold that simply won't go away or a series of colds. ("I can't believe that I caught six colds last winter.")

One of the secondary symptoms of chronic sinusitis is fatigue. Pressure from the sinuses cause cranial faults (a topic that will be covered later). Frequent infections cause the immune system to be overworked, which is very fatiguing. Also, sinusitis is a symptom of other things that have gone wrong with your physiology. It can be the result of allergies, poor diet, poor hydration or chemical toxicity—all of which can cause fatigue.

You need to keep your sinuses clear and your ostea open. Antibiotics for sinus infections don't address the cause of the problem. It's a lot like having a pile of open garbage and a problem with flies. If you spray insecticide, you'll kill the flies, but they always return, because the garbage is still there and flies like garbage. The spray will eventually wear off and succeeding generations of flies will be more immune to your spray. If you want to be rid of the flies, you have to get rid of the garbage. The same is true if you take antibiotics for your sinus infections. But if your sinuses stay full, you'll keep getting infections. The bacteria will become increasingly resistant to the antibiotics; thus, getting rid of each succeeding infection will become more difficult. You have to clear the mucous from the sinuses.

Sinuses that are full of mucous are not well protected by the immune system. They are warm and moist, and they have plenty of nutrients for microorganisms to feed on. The bloodstream and its immune defenses do not reach the material in the packed sinuses. Bacteria grow very easily in them. It's a lot like having a petrie dish up your nose.

Repeated bouts of antibiotic therapy for sinusitis can undermine your health. You may develop problems with yeast, allergies, poor digestion and repeated infections. These topics will be covered in the second half of the book.

Saline irrigation can reduce pain and swelling in the sinuses and nasal passages. Mix one cup of lukewarm water with 1/4 to 1/2 teaspoon of sea salt and a pinch of baking soda. Use 1/2 cup of the mixture for each nostril. Pour a little of the solution into the palm of one hand. Pinch one nostril shut and sniff the solution into your nose, one nostril at a time. The solution will run out of both nostrils and out of your mouth. This is not a lot of fun, but it will help your sinuses. Finish by blowing your nose. Irrigation is unpleasant, but it will help unplug the ostea and allow the sinuses to drain, reducing pressure and improving resistance to infection.

Sinuses are often worse in winter when they are exposed to hot, dry, indoor heat. Using a room humidifier will help keep sinuses moist and healthy. Make absolutely certain that you clean the humidifier and change the water twice each week. If you do not clean it, the humidifier may become a breeding ground for mold and you will become much, much worse.

Steam is very helpful to sinusitis sufferers. Long, hot showers, going into a steam bath or simply boiling water and inhaling the vapor through your nose will help the sinuses to drain.

Drinking plenty of water is also important. Sinuses are auxiliary elimination organs. Wastes that cannot get out of your body through the kidney or bowel will seep through mucous membranes. Drinking plenty of water will help you to eliminate waste efficiently, without plugging up your sinuses. You should have eight, eight-ounce glasses of water each day. Many sinus sufferers improve simply by drinking more water.

It would be worth your while to purchase a HEPA filter. HEPA is an acronym for high efficiency particulate arrestor. This is a freestanding air filter that will filter particles as small as 0.1 microns. It will also filter nearly 95% of all particles larger than 0.3 microns. Dust, mold and pollen particles are all larger than 0.3 microns. A HEPA filter will take a lot of the pollution, allergens and particulate matter out of the air, making the air cleaner and less irritating to the sinuses.

If you have forced-air heating, you may consider having the ducts cleaned. You'll be surprised at what comes out of your ductwork. Dust, mold and mites, all of which contribute to sinus problems and allergies, can be removed by cleaning the ducts. This is especially important if you have central air-conditioning. Mold frequently grows in the ducts of buildings with central air-conditioning.

Never sniff mucous back into your nose. Always blow it out. Sniffing plugs the ostea and increases your sinus pressure. Also, if you smoke, quit. Smokers are much more prone to sinus trouble than nonsmokers.

Bringing your sinusitis under control may eliminate your fatigue. If you suffer from sinusitis, pay particular attention to the sections about nutrition, bowel ecology and allergies as you read through the book.

Water

The adult human body is about 56% fluid. Individual cells contain between 70% and 85% water. Water is necessary for proper elimination of wastes and for good lymphatic flow.

Many people think that the body produces urine to get rid of excess water. Actually, the body produces urine in order to get rid of small amounts of solid waste. It uses water, which is precious to it, to get rid of these wastes.

When patients are told to drink eight, eight-ounce glasses of water each day, they usually say, "If I drank that much water, I'd live in the bathroom." If this is you, it means that you really need the water. Your body is holding onto waste products, waiting for you to have enough sense to drink water so it can get rid of the wastes.

Inadequate water intake decreases the lymphatic circulation, causing poor tissue oxygenation and waste removal. Waste products that should be carried away from the cell by the lymphatic system stay in the vicinity of the cell. You sit there marinating in your own waste products. Of course you're fatigued.

Not drinking enough water can cause constipation. The large intestine is the final five feet of the digestive tract. It produces no enzymes and absorbs few nutrients. The one thing that is absorbed in the large intestine is water. If a person is not properly hydrated, more water is absorbed from the large intestine than would be if the person drank plenty of water. This makes the stool dry and hard, resulting in constipation.

Constipation causes fatigue. The intestinal lymph nodes of someone suffering from chronic constipation are full of bacteria. This can contribute to leaky gut, dysbiosis and to immune system problems, all of which contribute to fatigue and even more serious health problems.

People with constipation often take fiber. Fiber increases the bulk of the stool and stimulates the digestive tract to move faster. If, however, the individual taking the fiber needs water, the stool becomes dry and hard and is not easily eliminated. It's a paradox: taking fiber laxatives can actually make constipation worse.

Your very first concern if you are constipated is whether or not you are getting enough water. Very often increasing water intake "cures" constipation. Fiber is also important if you want to bring constipation under control, but don't take fiber supplements. Get your fiber from eating plenty of fresh fruits and vegetables. Simply drinking water and eating fruits and vegetables cures most cases of constipation. If it does not, then there may be a problem with dysbiosis, hydrochloric acid, enzymes or the thyroid. These topics will be covered later.

Water quality is an important issue. The Environmental Protection Agency (EPA) has warned that the water in many areas is not fit to drink. If water quality is bad enough for the government to notice, it must be pretty bad. In 1995 a lot of people in Milwaukee became sick from bacteria that was not removed from their municipal water supply. Lead from old pipes often finds its way into tap water. This has been a big problem in the Chicago area. Drinking tap water may not be a good idea.

There is a lot of controversy about what kind of water is best. Spring water is very rich in minerals, especially iron and calcium. Unfortunately, much of the water is polluted with pesticides and industrial waste. Every so often you hear about an inordinate number of people in the same area dying of cancer. Frequently, chemicals in their water supply are to blame.

There are labs that will test your water for various pollutants. There are also kits you can buy to test the water yourself. National Testing Lab, Inc. in Cleveland, Ohio will test your water for heavy metals, pesticides and other contaminants for a modest fee. Their phone number is 800-458-3330.

Testing and filtering tap water is a good idea. City tap water has a lot of chlorine and fluorine in it. Even the government says not all tap water is safe.

There are activated carbon and reverse osmosis filters. This is an oversimplification, but activated carbon is good for removing organic materials, such as chemicals and pesticides. Reverse osmosis filters are good for removing metals such as lead and mercury. There are also filters that combine reverse osmosis and activated carbon. Make sure you change the filtering element when you're supposed to. Otherwise you may be adding pollutants to your drinking water.

There is a nonprofit organization that rates water filters called the National Sanitation Foundation or NSF. (NSF—I'm sure their checks don't bounce, they just have an unfortunate acronym.) NSF can be reached at:

P.O. Box 1468

Ann Arbor, Michigan 48106

When choosing a water filter, you can have your water tested, then choose the appropriate NSF-rated filter. If the filter you want to buy does not have an NSF rating, you can have the water tested before and after filtration.

Some people buy bottled distilled water. Proponents of distilled water claim that it is relatively pollution free. Critics say that it has no minerals and is not natural. If you place a cell into distilled water, it will explode. Another problem is that volatile pollutants (with a lower boiling point than water) can get distilled right in with the water.

There is bottled spring water for sale. Some of it is good; some of it is not. There are no controls over the quality of bottled water. You could start your own bottled water company with your tap and some jugs. Although, as of this writing, the government is just beginning to tighten up on the labeling rules for bottled water.

Water quality is important, but don't let worrying about your water keep you from drinking enough of it. Not consuming enough water can cause fatigue, constipation and even sinus trouble. You should drink at least eight, eight-ounce glasses of water each day.

General Nutrition

Vitamins are frequently recommended in health food stores to people who suffer from fatigue. Convenience stores sell "energy packs" consisting of three or four different vitamins, promising to give whoever takes them more energy.

Patients frequently ask what vitamin is good for fatigue. Taking vitamins, however, does not guarantee you more energy. In order for a vitamin to do you any good, you must need it.

You don't take a vitamin to make a specific physiologic change, like you would take a drug. You take aspirin for a headache, an antibiotic for an infection, diazide for blood pressure and so on. Taking vitamins to target specific health problems, like you take drugs, is not usually effective. People take vitamin C for their immune system, vitamin B for stress, vitamin E for sexual performance and so on. Vitamins are not meant to be taken that way. They work in combination with each other. Whole foods usually contain vitamins in their proper combinations. Eating whole, natural food is the best way to ensure good nutritional balance.

If there is a need for a particular vitamin, or an extreme deficiency, taking that vitamin will create what seems like a miracle. One person will take a vitamin B complex and become energetic. Another will take it and feel no effects at all. The first person needed vitamin B, the second did not. A vitamin is not effective unless there is a deficiency, even a slight one. If you are tired, and you need vitamin B, it will help you. If your fatigue is due to something else, you can take a pound of vitamin B and it won't make any difference.

Vitamin supplementation is often necessary. Because of mechanized agriculture, produce is often lacking in trace nutrients. A lifetime of poor eating habits, chemical exposure, drug therapies and other assaults on the body make vitamin supplementation necessary. Taking vitamins like they're drugs to target ailments is not always an effective strategy. Supplementation is just what the word implies: You augment a diet of nutrient-rich foods. Most of your vitamins should be gotten from good food: You supplement to help you in deficient areas. Some people are deficient in a lot of nutrients, and will benefit by taking lots of different vitamins. Others will find that a diet of whole foods supplies them with all of the vitamins and minerals they need.

It is true that someone fighting a cold may benefit from vitamin C, someone under stress may benefit from vitamin B, and someone with libido problems may benefit from vitamin E. People suffering from allergies and extreme fatigue have been helped by taking large doses of nutrients. However, **nutritional therapy is not like drug therapy.** There is an interrelationship among nutrients. Balance is as important, if not more important, than absolute amounts. In fact, taking too much of the wrong vitamin may aggravate your problem. Skill and an understanding of physiology and nutrition are needed to effectively use nutritional supplementation to improve your health.

Let's say, for example, that you tend to have bladder infections. You read that vitamin C is good for immune system problems and infections, and you take large doses of it. If you are vitamin A deficient (which may cause the membrane of the bladder to be more susceptible to infection), and if your urine tends to be acidic, taking large doses of vitamin C may make you worse.

Which vitamin will help with fatigue? The answer is simple: the one you are most deficient in. Nutrition and physiology are very complex. There are thousands of biochemical reactions going on in the body all of the time. Vitamins and minerals make these reactions possible. Even slight deficiencies in nutrients can affect the body's biochemistry. Often nothing is medically wrong, except for fatigue or another vague symptom.

You may notice Ed in accounting. He's the guy who used to shuffle through the office, head down, eyes at half-mast. Suddenly Ed seems to have a new lease on life. He takes up squash, bungi jumping and mountain climbing, and gets a 19-year-old girlfriend. You're impressed because Ed's 96 (and he doesn't even use Amour-all on his dashboard.) You ask him his secret, and he shows you his new stress vitamin that is packed with antioxidants, ginseng, bee pollen, Chinese herbs and some kind of extract made from hummingbird testicles. Ed tells you all of this at his villa in Hawaii, during a recruitment meeting for a multilevel marketing scheme to sell this vitamin. He got in early, at the top of the pyramid, so he earns more than the gross national product of several small countries. You figure that you could use a little more energy and the money sounds good, so you try it. You begin by investing $600 for some of the product and the basic sales kit. After you start taking the supplement you get sick to your stomach and break out in purple spots. Ed says not to worry, it's just part of the detox. You become a little concerned when the detox lasts for three and a half years. Your spots don't go away, and in three and a half years you've only managed to sell two bottles of the stuff (the purple spots are a real deterrent to sales). It just doesn't work.

If the guy at the health food store, the article in Prevention magazine or Ed picks a vitamin that you are deficient in, and you try it, you'll feel better. If it doesn't have anything you need, it won't do you much good. Ed's body needed extract of hummingbird testicles, and yours didn't.

Even if you take a vitamin that your body needs, this does not guarantee that you'll feel better. You may have health issues that override the small improvement that taking a necessary vitamin may provide. You may read an article that tells you that vitamin B complex reduces stress and increases energy. You may even have a friend that tried it and had good results. It is possible for you to take the vitamin B and not experience much of a change in how you feel. Either you didn't need vitamin B, or you had so many other health issues that taking vitamin B didn't help you very much.

There are thousands of biochemical reactions going on in the body all of the time. Vitamins and minerals make these reactions possible. Nerve impulses that make feeling and movement possible, enzyme production that makes digestion possible, hormone production, waste removal and even muscle movement are made possible by thousands of chemical reactions that are dependent on balanced biochemistry made possible by proper nutrition. Chemical balance—which makes it possible for the cells of the body to have energy, make their products, eliminate waste and reproduce—is dependent on good nutrition.

It is not as if these reactions completely shut down with an improper diet. If that were true, there would not be an overpopulation problem. We have the capacity to store most nutrients. Our bodies also have a way of prioritizing the use of nutrients. The brain, heart and kidneys are kept running at the expense of other bodily functions when nutrients are in short supply.

A body in a poor nutritional state does not necessarily become diseased in the sense that traditional Western doctors, trained to find pathology, would notice. Pathology usually doesn't develop until many years of neglect. Neglecting health leads to a variety of subclinical complaints such as: fatigue, joint pain, frequent colds, allergies, sinusitis, rashes, hives, dry skin, depression, headaches and other health problems.

We are now in the third generation of junk food. Fast food and empty calories have been a way of life since the 1950s. Pollution is getting worse and our soil is becoming depleted of trace nutrients. Nutritionally depleted parents are having children that are even more nutritionally depleted. As time goes on, nutritional reserves are less for each succeeding generation. Some vague, chronic complaints are now becoming named disease entities, such as chronic fatigue syndrome, fibromyalgia, attention deficit disorder, and hyperactivity in children. It may seem to you that there are more chronically ill children. There are children who have had several courses of antibiotics before the age of five, are obese, have trouble paying attention in school and have behavioral problems. Poor health seems to be increasing.

It's always amusing when someone from the medical community is quoted in the paper or on the news saying something like, "Vitamins do not cure disease!" It's an absurd statement when you consider the fact that vitamins cure the disease of vitamin deficiency.

The symptoms of vitamin deficiency are many and varied. Unfortunately, many doctors are well versed in pharmacology, pathology and surgery, but know less about normal physiology than Gallagher knows about decorum or Bill Clinton knows about infantry training.

Studies have been done to see if vitamin E can help arthritis. There are modest results, but the vitamin is never incorporated into regular treatment. What should be done is a study of arthritics who are vitamin E deficient and see how many of them are helped. Better yet, do a complete nutritional analysis of some arthritics and create individual programs for them and see how many of those people find relief.

Unfortunately, it is unlikely that such a study will be performed because scientific studies focus only on single issues. This is why we get such bizarre and conflicting nutritional information from the scientific community. We are not petrie dishes. Human beings are so complex,. Our biochemistry involves so many variables that tests involving a single aspect of nutrition do not yield good results.

Consider a recent study researching cholesterol. Researchers were bound and determined to prove that cholesterol consumption led to high blood cholesterol, arterial sclerosis and heart disease. They spent years studying people and their cholesterol consumption and compiled statistical information about cholesterol and heart disease. They came to the conclusion that they set out to prove: Cholesterol consumption leads to high blood cholesterol and eventually leads to plaquing of the arterial walls and heart disease. The announcement of the results had us all watching our cholesterol.

When significant numbers of people did not respond to low cholesterol diets, a drug was created to control the "disease" of high cholesterol. People started taking these drugs with no real evidence that they will increase the length of their life.

Here's the logic: high cholesterol consumption leads to high blood cholesterol, which leads to heart disease. Eat low cholesterol and avoid heart disease. OOPS, not everyone eating low cholesterol can bring their blood cholesterol down—let's make a drug.

The whole thing is ludicrous. The fact that the liver makes cholesterol was ignored. The fact that carbohydrate metabolism is related to cholesterol production was ignored. Liver function, a lack of essential fatty acids, vitamin deficiency, chemicals and refined carbohydrate affect cholesterol levels, and need to be considered. High cholesterol is not a disease, but a symptom of something else that is wrong, either with the diet or the functioning of the liver or the digestive system.

It's like the story of the Harvard researcher who was working with frogs. He'd yell and slam a rolled newspaper near the frog. The startled frog would jump. The researcher made the frog jump several times. He took notes, plotted his results on a graph and averaged them out. He found that, on average, the frog jumped 20 feet.

He then cut a leg off of the frog and repeated the experiment. He yelled and slammed the rolled newspaper behind the animal. On average the frog jumped 15 feet.

The researcher repeated the experiment after cutting off another of the frog's legs. On average the frog could jump only 10 feet.

He cut off a third leg, made a very loud noise by yelling and slamming the newspaper. The poor frog struggled, but did manage to jump five feet.

After cutting off the last of the frog's legs off, the researcher tried to get it to jump. He yelled louder and louder. He slammed the paper harder and harder, but the frog just lay there. The researcher came to the conclusion that removing all of the legs made the animal hard of hearing.

The point is that research only offers a narrow range of information, which is open to interpretation. There really isn't much difference between the cholesterol study and the research involving the frog.

I realize that many of you are indignant that the researcher caused the frog so much suffering in the name of science. I felt the same way and tried to contact him, but was unsuccessful. He was pummeled to death with organic carrots by a vegetarian street gang, the Soys in the 'Hood.

Drugs are much more widely researched than vitamins. One of the reasons is that drugs can be patented, vitamins cannot. The huge profits pharmaceutical companies realize from drug sales are just not possible with vitamins. Drugs can cause massive changes in physiology that more natural substances are incapable of causing, making research on drugs more cut and dried. (Come to think of it, there are natural substances that cause massive changes in physiology, but they're illegal.)

There is a research-driven mythology in this country. The television news likes to use little health tidbits released by researchers.

Unfortunately they don't tell you any of the details of the study performed, only the conclusion. For instance, recently a study was performed on children and whether or not sugar was involved with hyperactivity. The children in the experiment were put on additive-free diets and given a measured dose of sugar. The researchers came to the conclusion that sugar did not affect hyperactivity. Of course the argument can be made that having the children on additive-free diets made them less prone to be hyperactive, but that idea was left out of the news report. The news only reported "Sugar has no effect on hyperactive children." They created a myth. If our frog experiment was reported on the television news, we'd hear, "Frogs hear with their legs. Film at eleven." When better research is done and comes to better conclusions, we'll hear that. This is why we keep getting conflicting information about health. You are told to eat margarine, then you are told not to eat margarine. It's very confusing. You can't make up your mind so you keep waiting for another news report to straighten things out. Unfortunately, the news doesn't exist to inform you. It exists to entertain you enough to keep you watching so the sponsors can sell you hemorrhoid cream and diet cola.

The type of research being done in this country, the philosophy of our doctors and a general laziness on our part, are why we have sickness care instead of health care. We fight cancer, heart disease and other diseases; we don't promote health. While it's true that there are new attempts to get Americans to change their lifestyles, these attempts are feeble compared to the efforts that go into developing new drugs and technology to battle disease.

The biggest health problem in America is not cancer or heart disease. We are not lacking in new drugs or technology. The biggest health problem is the fact that so many Americans are tired all of the time. **One of the major causes of the epidemic of fatigue in this country is poor nutrition.**

24

If you solve the problem of fatigue early in life, you will reduce the chances of serious disease later in life.

Inadequate intake of vitamins and minerals can exist for several reasons. Eating a nutrient-deficient, refined diet, alcoholism or drug abuse, poor digestion or absorption, chemical pollution from pesticides and food additives, and even genetic defects can all lead to poor nutritional status.

It is preferable to get your vitamins from nutritious food than to get them from pills. However, severe deficiency may make it necessary to take supplements. There are clues that tell you whether you need a particular vitamin.

For instance, if you have been spending years eating a lot of sugar, white flour and not eating whole grains, you probably need vitamin B complex, vitamin C and minerals. People who need vitamin B complex frequently get headaches that feel like a band around their head, and they may have problems staying asleep at night.

If you lack vitamin B6, you won't remember your dreams. If you take B6 and it doesn't help, you may need to take the active form, pyridoxyl-5-phosphate. If you only get help from the active form of B6, it probably means that you need magnesium. When you are outside with a group of people and it seems like you are the only one being bitten by insects, you probably need niacin and riboflavin (vitamin B3 and vitamin B2). People needing folic acid often confuse right and left or transpose letters and numbers when writing. Folic acid is a common deficiency because it is destroyed by cooking.

One of the best ways to tell if you need zinc is to taste zinc sulfate liquid. This is available in a product called Zinc Tally, which is made by Metagenics. Taste a capful of the liquid. If you are extremely deficient in zinc, the liquid will be tasteless. If you have a slight deficiency, it will have a slight bitter taste. If you do not need zinc, the liquid will taste bitter and strong. (The word horrible falls far short of the description of the way this tastes to people who don't need zinc.) Other signs of zinc deficiency are white spots on the finger nails and patches of dry skin.

People with nails that are brittle and crack frequently need trace minerals. These people may also benefit from a supplement that includes all eight essential amino acids. These deficiencies are often the result of an underproduction of hydrochloric acid in the stomach, known as hypochlorhydra.

Excessive body odor or sweaty feet is often an indication of a need for magnesium. (If your feet smell and your nose runs, you're built upside down.) Also, taking magnesium and B6 can reduce the tendency to get kidney stones.

If you have dry skin, muscle fatigue and dandruff or if you crave greasy foods, you probably need essential fatty acids. Also, if you take aspirin frequently, and it is a good pain reliever for you, essential fatty acids may help you to get by with less aspirin.

The best way to get your vitamins is still from whole food. Vitamin supplementation can get you over some rough spots, but is not a substitute for a proper diet.

Food

Everything the body does is a chemical reaction, and food is the raw material for these reactions. Your body burns carbohydrate as fuel. Fat is stored, and is used as fuel in times when food is scarce. Fat is also important to the endocrine and the immune system. Protein is used as structural material and to give osmotic pressure to the blood. Protein is also used as a raw material for enzymes, which are proteins that cause chemical reactions without being changed by the reaction; they are organic catalysts. Protein aids in immunity in the blood and helps the nervous system to work. Vitamins and minerals in your diet act as cofactors to enzymes, sort of like the ignition key in an automobile. They enable the enzymes to function.

Carbohydrates come in two forms—sugar and complex carbohydrates. Sugar is a small molecule. Simple sugars have six carbon molecules. Think of a sugar molecule as a boxcar. A disaccharide is two linked boxcars. Starch, or complex carbohydrate, is like a train, with dozens of boxcars linked together.

Similarly, protein is a long molecule, like a freight train. The smaller molecules making up the boxcars of the protein train are called amino acids. Eight of the 22 amino acids are essential, which means that they cannot be produced by the body and must be eaten in the diet.

Fats are put together a little differently than carbohydrates and proteins. The base molecule for fat is the triglyceride. It is a three-pronged molecule, with glycerol as a base. Attached to each of the prongs of the molecule is a long molecule called a fatty acid.

Sterols are another form of fat that have an entirely different structure than triglycerides. Sterols are ringed molecules. The best known of these is cholesterol. Sterols are important in the formation of hormones.

Digestion is the process of taking each of these large fat, protein and carbohydrate molecules, breaking them down into small molecules and transporting them into the blood stream. Protein is broken down into amino acids. Complex carbohydrates are broken down into sugars. Fat is broken down into fatty acids and glycerin. The small molecules can then be absorbed by the body and used by the cells as raw material.

Sugar

Eating refined sugar damages your health and energy.
Many people increase their energy simply by giving up refined sugar. Eating sweets changes the pH of your digestive system, making it more alkaline. Intestinal pH is very important to your health. The enzymes that digest your food are pH dependent. The bacteria that live in your large intestine are sensitive to changes in pH. Too much sugar is harmful to digestion and nutrient absorption.

In your intestines, there is a delicate balance of nature between bacteria and yeast. If you eat a lot of sugar, you create an environment that favors yeast growth. Too much yeast can cause a lot of problems. You may tend to bloat or get tired when you eat. You may develop allergies. Many women become prone to vaginal yeast infections. Ironically, yeast overgrowth can make you crave sugar.

Eating refined sugar is also hard on the endocrine system. It puts stress on the pancreas and on the adrenal glands, causing fatigue. If you are tired and you eat a lot of sugar, give it up and you'll feel better.

Sugar tends to be addictive. Eating it causes a sudden increase in your blood sugar, which scares the heck out of your pancreas. Your pancreas hasn't evolved since Neolithic times and hasn't the foggiest idea of what a Twix bar is. You have the pancreas of a caveman, and it responds to the increase in your blood sugar as if you'd just eaten a bushel of potatoes. It makes enough insulin to respond to a future need. Unfortunately, the increase in blood sugar from the Twix bar you just ate is short-lived. You end up with extra insulin circulating through your bloodstream. Your body interprets this as wanting more sugar. The cravings are pretty strong, and many people have trouble giving up sugar.

Bringing sugar cravings under control is easier than most people realize. Many can usually bring their cravings under control within a day. The key is not to go more than two hours without snacking. If lunch is at noon and dinner at six, eat a piece of fruit at two and at four. Fruit is your snack of choice because it has natural sugar and will curb your craving. Chewing your food thoroughly also will help to control sugar cravings. Chewing improves digestion and absorption of nutrients bringing hunger and food cravings under control.

Problems with digestion and absorption may make it difficult to give up sugar. Refined sugar is very easily absorbed. It is much easier to digest and absorb than protein or even whole grains. Even people with digestion and absorption problems absorb sugar easily. People who do not digest protein or other nutrients very well, crave sugar. Unconsciously they understand that they will get *some* nutrient out of that Hershey bar. They may even be aware that they don't feel very well when they eat wholesome foods. You see this a lot in older people. They don't care much for meat, but they love desserts.

As people get older, they produce less hydrochloric acid for digestion, making it more difficult to digest protein. Some think this is why people get osteoarthritis. The body needs protein to sustain life. The brain, kidneys, heart and other vital organs all need protein. When there is a lack of protein (in this case because of a problem digesting protein), the body has a priority system deciding where the protein goes. It will steal the protein from less important areas, such as joint surfaces, for use in areas that are vital for survival.

Joint movement is not as important as kidney, heart or brain function. (Well, maybe joint movement is more important than brain function in congressmen, career government bureaucrats and certain NFL draft picks.) In order to survive, the body sacrifices ease of movement, which is a luxury compared to these other functions.

Allergies can also make it difficult to give up sugar. Often someone who can't give up sugar has an allergy to either corn (and therefore corn syrup, one of the more common sweeteners), cane sugar or even chocolate. People who are allergic to a food tend to be addicted to it, much the same way an alcoholic is addicted. In fact, Theron Randolph (noted allergist and a man who can be considered the founder of clinical ecology), calls alcoholism the ultimate food allergy.

Eating refined sugar makes the adrenal glands overwork in order to keep up the blood sugar level. Refined sugar overworks the pancreas, and causes major problems with digestion and with the general health of the digestive tract. Refined sugar creates nutrient deficiencies and causes fatigue in so many different ways that you cannot reasonably expect to feel energetic unless you eliminate refined sugar from your diet.

The Importance of Whole Grains

Because of Americans' paranoia about fat, pasta is now being lauded as a health food. Pasta is low in fat, but most pasta is made with refined white flour. Filling up on white bread and noodles because they are low in fat is a lot like eating road apples because they don't have cyanide. Just because one thing that isn't healthy isn't present in a food, doesn't automatically make that food a good one. Two-by-fours are low in fat, but you wouldn't want to eat one with a mess of marinara sauce, would you?

Eating refined white flour products causes some of the same problems that eating sugar causes. Refined white flour is broken down and absorbed very quickly, much like sugar. It also causes the same changes in bowel pH as sugar does.

In nature, anything that contains complex carbohydrates also contains some vitamin B, vitamin E and fiber. Interestingly, B vitamins aid in carbohydrate metabolism. When you eat whole grains, you are automatically consuming the vitamins you need to process them.

Some refined products are labeled enriched, which is a great piece of doublespeak that would make George Orwell proud. Enriching means that the manufacturer takes all of the B vitamins, vitamin E, essential fatty acids and fiber out of the grain, then puts back some of the B vitamins. Let me borrow $100. I'll give you $5 back and tell you that I enriched your money.

Let's say that someone stole your BMW (Oops, this is the '90s, I mean your Lexus.) The police find it. The thieves have stripped the car completely; they've taken the stereo, the cellular phone, the leather seats, the quarter panels, the tires and the engine. They even took your toll booth change and your Barry Manilow CD. The thieves decided that they wanted to drive the frame. They put in mismatched tires, a bucket seat from an old AMC Pacer, a gas tank from a 1973 Pinto and an engine from an old DeSoto. The door is being held closed with a bungi cord

30

and your Barry Manilow CD is being used for an ashtray. The police call you and tell you that they've located your enriched automobile. That loaf of white bread has been enriched in a similar manner.

Eat foods the way nature created them. There is a good deal of misinformation circulating about nutrition. People tend to think in terms of RDAs and absolute amounts of nutrients. Most of the vitamins were discovered in the 1930s when chemical know-how wasn't very sophisticated. For example, as far as the government is concerned, ascorbic acid is vitamin C; but a food that is high in vitamin C has much more in it than just ascorbic acid. Food containing vitamin C complex has bioflavenoids, vitamin K and other nutrients. Eating food that is high in vitamin C is different from taking ascorbic acid.

Vitamin B complex is present in foods that contain complex carbohydrates. The B vitamins in these foods exist in very definite proportions to each other and to certain synergistic minerals that enable them to be absorbed by your body. These important combinations are never taken into consideration when manufacturers enrich their products.

The chemistry of the living cell and the human body is much more complex than the chemistry that takes place in a lab or a beaker. Biomolecules work like little factories or fine machinery. You can give a chemist a Rolex watch, and he or she can analyze it and tell you how much gold, glass, quartz and other materials are in it. You can take the same watch and smash it with a hammer and, from the chemist's point of view, nothing has changed. Cellulose and starch have the same chemical formula. Chemically, there is no difference between wood and a potato, except how the molecule is arranged. Many things added to foods, put there by manufacturers as nutrients, are as useful to the body as wood.

Complex carbohydrates in nature always contain fiber. It is cellulose from the cell walls of plants. You cannot digest and absorb it. Other nutrients adhere to fiber and are absorbed more slowly than they would be if there were no fiber in the meal. It sort of makes your meal time released. The gradual absorption of whole grain is not nearly as much of a burden on your pancreas as the rapid absorption of refined grains. White bread and pasta are rapidly absorbed, causing the blood sugar to increase, stressing the pancreas.

The fiber in whole grains also cuts down on the number of calories and fat you absorb from your food. It makes your bowel healthy and reduces your chances of getting cancer by increasing bowel motility and reducing the toxicity of the bowel. Normal bowel bacteria feed on fiber, so a diet that is high in fiber helps keep the bowel healthy. White bread has no fiber.

You own the body of a prehistoric hunter-gatherer. Food technology has changed faster than your body's ability to adapt to those changes. Your body has not adapted to eating starch or sugar that is not consumed with vitamins and fiber. Sugar or complex carbohydrates eaten in their natural state, with the fiber, are absorbed slowly. White flour and sugar are absorbed more quickly than anything your prehistoric ancestors had.

Eating refined foods makes the pancreas produce insulin at a very rapid rate. The pancreas overproduces insulin and causes a hypoglycemic state. You end up with all of that extra insulin, and nothing for it to do except lower the blood sugar, making your crave more sweets or starch.

These blood sugar swings are hard on your endocrine system. They are stressful. Physiologically, your body doesn't know the difference between this stress and having Atilla the Hun for a boss, a cheating spouse or a certified letter from Adolph Q. Sphincter of the IRS suggesting you show up at their offices with your 1989-1994 income tax records. The stress of blood sugar swings is one reason why refined foods cause fatigue.

32

The stress of eating incorrectly is as tiring as the stress of worrying, physically exhausting yourself or not sleeping. Your endocrine system simply doesn't know the difference.

People in primitive societies who are suddenly exposed to modern diets experience a dramatic increase in health problems. Johnathan Wright, in his book Dr. Wright's Guide to Healing With Nutrition, has several examples of the deterioration of primitive people after adopting a modern diet. The most notable change in their diet was an increase in sugar and other refined carbohydrates. One example in Dr. Wright's book is the Eskimos living in Northern Canada. It is taken from an article entitled "When the Eskimo Comes to Town" by Otto Schaefer, which appeared in the November/December 1971 issue of Nutrition Today. The Eskimos studied had no exposure to civilization until the 1940s. Within 10 years of the dietary change, the number of diabetics tripled. Five times as many men over 40 developed diseases of the arteries. Gallbladder surgery, which was never necessary for these people, became common. Teenagers developed acne, and some women developed breast cancer, maladies which were unheard of prior to 1940 and the Eskimos' change in diet.

Sugar and other refined carbohydrates undermine your health and energy level, much the same way that it destroyed the health of the Canadian Eskimos. The only difference is that we have had this diet for so long that we aren't aware of the damage it is causing.

Sugar and starch cravings can be brought under control by snacking between meals. Eating every two or three hours will help you avoid the drops in blood sugar that make these empty calories so appealing. If eating frequently doesn't work, you may have problems with food allergies, digestion or yeast. Vitamin B or exercise can sometimes help keep you from craving refined foods.

Fresh Fruits and Vegetables

You should have a minimum of four cups of fresh vegetables and three pieces of fruit every day. Have more, if you like. Fruit and vegetables are high in bulk and fiber and will improve your digestion, speed up your bowel transit time, nourish your normal bowel flora and decrease the toxicity in your colon. Your health and energy will increase and your chances for developing bowel cancer will decrease.

If you are constipated, there is a very good chance that your lack of energy is linked to your bowel. It is very important that you eat enough fresh produce. Drinking plenty of water and eating plenty of fruits and vegetables will cure most cases of constipation.

Digesting food takes a lot of energy. Those people with inefficient digestive systems use more energy than those who digest well. The bulk, fiber and enzymatic help from fresh fruits and vegetables will improve your digestion and eliminate a major source of fatigue.

Fruits and vegetables are also rich in vitamins and minerals and low in calories. Nutritional deficiency is a major cause of fatigue. Those who don't eat fresh produce often suffer from fatigue due to a lack of certain nutrients. Eating fresh fruits and vegetables provides plenty of nutrients, makes the body's chemistry function optimally and increases energy.

Raw Foods

Americans eat too much cooked food. Food that is cooked requires all of the digestive enzymes to be produced by the body. Cooked food is harder to digest than raw food. Raw fruits and vegetables contain enzymes that aid digestion

Cooking also destroys some vitamins. Heat destroys thiamin (B1), riboflavin (B2) and pantothenic acid (B5). Pantothenic acid is destroyed by heat in the presence of an acid or alkali. It is stable in neutral solutions.

34

Vitamins B5 and B6 can be destroyed by light. Vitamin B12 and folic acid are easily oxidized to a form not usable by the body. Other vitamins can be destroyed by either alkaline or acid pH. Even exposure to light can destroy certain nutrients.

This is not to say that you should avoid cooked food. You should just try to eat some raw vegetables or fruit with every meal. Food is always best in its natural state.

Additives, Agribusiness and the Other Side of Poor Nutrition

Even if you are eating what you think is a good diet, you may not be getting enough of certain vitamins, and you may be consuming a lot of toxic substances. Your diet can be causing your fatigue without your being aware of it. **The average American consumes 10 pounds of food additives per year.** This is just additives that the food industry purposely puts in food. This doesn't count the insecticides, fungicides, herbicides and other chemicals used by farmers.

Processing, even simple cooking, decreases the nutritional value of food. Boiling leaches vitamins and minerals out of the food and into the cooking water. Certain vitamins are not stable to heat.

Food manufacturers and processors do not pay attention to the nutritional content of the foods they prepare. They are more concerned with taste, shelf life, texture and appearance. Processed food is a victory of form over substance.

A variety of chemicals are added to food to preserve it and to give it desirable texture, firmness and consistency. Sugar and fat are added to enhance the food's desirability and to mask the taste of the additives. There is even a chemical to help hide the taste of the other chemicals. The manufacturers want the consumer to perceive their products as real food that has the qualities we value in food, even if it is chemically laden and valueless. A little bit of chemical know-how and Voila! you have a "food" that can stay on your grocer's shelf until the Second Coming, and still be edible. (Well, sellable anyway; it probably never was edible.)

Thousands of years from now, archaeologists will find a package of Mostess Winkies in some ruins. The cakes will still be soft and edible (or at least not any less edible than they were when they were manufactured). Scientists will marvel at this discovery. Much will be said about our culture's ability to embalm food. Some of the scientists will postulate that the food was meant to be buried with kings to supply them with nutrients on their long trip to the underworld. The Winkies will be sold at auction for a small fortune, like wine found in ancient Roman ruins is sold today.

Many patients, after being advised about how harmful additives are, ask if frozen dinners are healthy. They see the labels on frozen foods and find them to be relatively chemical-free—for convenience foods. The problem is, that if these are eaten frequently, the diet becomes very deficient in vitamin C and most of the B vitamins.

Researchers at Rutgers University measured the levels of vitamin C in a frozen chicken pot pie. They couldn't find any. They then added a known amount of vitamin C to the thawed pie, refroze it and heated it two days later. They found that this process destroyed about 25% of the vitamin C.

Frozen foods, while having fewer chemicals than many other processed foods, tend to be vitamin deficient. It is not a good idea to have frozen dinners every day. Frozen food is, however, better for you than many of the additive-laden foods people eat every day.

Compare the bread that is sold to the American public to the bread that was consumed by primitive societies. It will give you an idea of how technology has undermined health. The ancient Egyptians developed the technique of grinding grain between two stones. The technique produced flour that could be made into a cohesive dough. Since that time, light-colored bread has been prized. The more of the bran that is removed, the whiter the bread. The light-colored bread of ancient times still had some of the bran and all of the wheat germ. Ancient societies did not have the technology to completely strip the nutrients from grain. We have that technology today. Modern white flour is completely striped of nutrients. It has none of the germ, which contains vitamin E and octocosinol. It has none of the bran, which contains the B vitamins and fiber.

Modern bakers were inconvenienced by the fact that the baking qualities of flour varied from batch to batch. Consistency between batches has been achieved by bleaching the flour with chlorine gas.

Bleached flour is a much more workable product for the mechanized food industry. Unfortunately, chlorine does more than bleach and mature the flour. It interacts with the other molecules in the flour, creating things like the chlorinated lipid, dichlorostearic acid. Another bleaching agent, nitrogen trichloride reacts with methionine residues and forms methionine sulfoximine, which can cause nervous seizures, similar to epilepsy. The chlorine also destroys any vitamin E that may be left in the flour.

Modern commercial bread frequently has added mono and diglycerides in order to make it soft. If you add a little potassium bromate, you can whip up the bread and cause it to rise in as little as two minutes. Never mind the fact that potassium bromate is a deadly poison; it's a small price to pay for increased production, efficiency and consistency between batches. Of course now our modern product has five chemicals added and all of the nutrients removed—and you're wondering why you're tired.

Here is the list of ingredients of a typical loaf of modern white bread: enriched all purpose flour, enzyme active soy preparation, salt, sugar, lard, skim milk powder, monoglycerides, diglycerides, calcium proprionate, yeast food (containing flour, salt calcium sulfate, ammonium chloride and potassium bromate), benzoyl peroxide, niacin, iron, tricalcium phosphate, potassium bromate, thiamine mononitrite and magnesium carbonate.

In exchange for the fiber, vitamin E, octocosinol and vitamin B complex removed from the bread, the manufacturer has added a half dozen chemicals and two B vitamins. The experts in charge of telling the American public about nutrition, after much debate, have decided to tell us to eat according to a food pyramid and to get plenty of grains. Unfortunately, they make no distinction between the garbage listed above and whole grains.

Look in Ruth Winters' Consumer's Dictionary of Food Additives to learn what some of the stuff that's been added to the bread is.

Mono and diglycerides: Used to maintain softness. Diglycerides are on the FDA list of food additives to be studied for possible mutagenic, teratogenic, subacute and reproductive effects. This is medicalese for birth defects, cancer and reproductive problems.

Calcium proprionate: Mold inhibitor, generally regarded as safe by the FDA.

Benzoyl peroxide: A bleaching agent; also skin irritant and possible allergen. Benzoyl peroxide is toxic if inhaled. Generally regarded as safe by the FDA. It's used in acne cream.

Tricalcium phosphate: An anticaking agent and a dietary supplement with no known toxicity.

Potassium bromate: Used to obtain a fine, spongelike quality in the bread. Legal allowance is 50 ppb (ppb = parts per billion). Very toxic when taken internally. Between two and four ounces of a 2% bromine solution can poison a child. Burns and skin irritation have been reported from its industrial uses. In 1980 the Ames test found potassium bromate to be a mutagen. The Ames test was developed by Dr. Bruce Ames, a biochemist at the University of California in the early 1970s. He developed the test using bacteria that reveals whether a chemical is a mutagen; that is, one that causes genetic changes in the bacteria. Almost all chemicals that are known carcinogens have also shown to be mutagenic on the Ames test. Whether the test can identify carcinogens is still controversial. This is much the same way the "Flat Earth Society" finds the idea that the world is round, controversial, or that the tobacco industry finds the link between smoking and lung cancer, controversial.

Magnesium carbonate: Generally regarded as safe.

Calcium sulfate: Plaster of Paris. (Helluva thing to find in bread, isn't it?) Calcium sulfate is used as a firming agent, yeast food and dough conditioner. Because it absorbs moisture and hardens quickly, its ingestion may result in intestinal obstruction. Mixed with flour, it has been used to kill rodents. Generally regarded as safe by the FDA.

Ammonium chloride: Dough conditioner and yeast food. Naturally occurring and generally regarded as safe by the FDA. Ammonium chloride can cause nausea, vomiting and acidosis in doses of 0.5-1.0 grams.

In a 110-pound batch of bread there is about 75 grams of additives, not counting the vitamins added to enrich the product. It's about three ounces of chemical, a little less than one gram per loaf. Some are harmful, some are not so harmful, according to the FDA. You many think that this is not a lot to consume; the FDA certainly doesn't. Unfortunately, the studies that allow the chemicals to be placed in food are done on animals, one chemical at a time. There are no studies on the cumulative effects of all of the additives. Also, this amount is not including the chemicals produced when the natural ingredients of the bread interact with the additives, such as dichlorostearic acid and methionine sulfoximine.

Let's say that you have this bread for lunch. You have a bologna sandwich, made with low-fat turkey bologna, because you're health conscious. You have a diet orange soda because you want to avoid sugar and caffeine, and you're watching your weight. You have a salad made of iceberg lettuce because the American Cancer Society finally got around to recommending fruits and vegetables after spending decades telling you that diet has nothing to do with cancer.

Your diet orange soda has aspartame (Nutrasweet), citric acid, sodium benzoate, gum acacia, natural flavors, glycerol, ester of wood rosin, yellow #6, brominated vegetable oil, and red #40. Winter's book *A Consumer's Dictionary of Food Additives* is an excellent resource for finding out what exactly the chemicals are in your food. Information about additives have been obtained form other sources as well, including David Steinman's book *Diet for a Poisoned Planet* and Kirk Hamilton's publication "Clinical Pearls." Let's take a look at some of these ingredients.

Aspartame: Sold under the brand names Nutrasweet and Equal. This was approved by the FDA for limited use, in crystalline form, in 1981. The approval came over the objections of a federal panel that wanted further testing to examine a possible link between brain cancer and aspartame. Indeed, there has been an increase in brain cancer since aspartame's approval. Some experts believe there may be a link between aspartame and headaches, anxiety attacks, memory loss, breathing difficulty, heart palpitations, nausea, seizures and blurred vision. Aspartame also raises the pH of urine, creating a tendency for the user to get bladder infections.

There have been some studies that seem to indicate that there is no connection between seizures and aspartame use; however, these have utilized the crystalline form of aspartame, given in a single dosage. Aspartame, when heated or in liquid, releases methanol, which is poisonous. Also, aspartame users take it in small doses throughout the day. There needs to be more studies, but these researchers have currently occupied themselves with studying hearing in frogs.

Sodium benzoate: A preservative that has been around for a long time. No known toxicity.

Gum acacia: Used to retard sugar crystallization. Also used as a foam stabilizer in soft drinks. Generally regarded as safe by the FDA. Gum acacia causes allergic reactions in some people.

Natural flavors: According to Ruth Winter's book, the FDA considers something natural if it involves only minimal processing, such as peeling homogenizing, baking and other things that can be done in the kitchen. Also, the food cannot have anything synthetic or any added chemicals. Beyond that, you don't know what these natural flavors are.

Ester of wood rosin: Wood rosin is the exudate from a living southern pine tree; it has no known toxicity. Ester is a compound formed from the rosin to reduce its allergy-causing properties

Yellow #6: Possible link to kidney and adrenal tumors. Yellow #6 has been banned in Norway and Sweden.

Brominated vegetable oil: Used as an emulsifier. The FDA has it on the suspect list. Bromates are highly toxic. They can cause death through kidney failure or nervous system problems. Bromates can inhibit the body's defenses.

Between two and four ounces of a 2% solution can poison a child. Also, severe allergic reactions have been reported. Brominated vegetable oil has also been found in human fat tissue, which means that the body stores this poison.

Red #40: Suspected carcinogen. Whenever you see a color followed by a number, avoid that food.

Your low-fat bologna has added: dextrose, hydrogenated milk protein, sodium phosphate, sodium erythrobate and sodium nitrite.

Dextrose: Corn sugar.

Hydrogenated milk protein: Generally regarded as safe by the FDA.

42

Sodium phosphate: Generally regarded as safe by the FDA.

Sodium erythrobate: An antioxidant with no known toxicity.

Sodium nitrite: Makes meat bright red and kills Clostridium Botulinum spores (botulism). Nitrite combines with natural stomach chemicals and chemicals in the food to form nitrosamines, which are **powerful carcinogens.**

Isn't it interesting that nitrites are known carcinogens. That's right, **known carcinogens,** not suspected, not just some suspicious tests. We know that nitrates create a chemical in the stomach that causes cancer. There isn't even a warning label on these products. The FDA has taken the view that nitrites kill botulism spores, and there is nothing to take the place of nitrites. Still, it seems odd that the FDA wouldn't have the manufacturers warn the parents who give their children bologna sandwiches and hot dogs for lunch that they may be giving their children cancer. I'm sure that the processed meat industry, being a $125 billion per year industry, had nothing to do with the FDA's decision. This is the same FDA that banned tryptophan because of one brand that was contaminated. This is the same FDA that raided, with guns drawn, the office of Dr. Jonathan Wright, M.D. Wright's crime? Using injectable vitamin B which did not have chemical preservatives in it. You may have to do a little homework and protect yourself with respect to food additives, considering the fact that you can't buy tryptophan, an essential amino acid, a natural substance, but you can get brominated vegetable oil and nitrites in your food.

The FDA raid on Dr. Wright's office might be worth mentioning here. It is, in a way, a health issue. It will contrast the permissiveness the FDA has with food additives to how it approaches those who are interested in natural health care. If it were shot in Hollywood, the scene at Dr. Wright's Tahoma Clinic in Kent, Washington on May 6, 1992 would have been titled "Rambo Meets the Three Stooges." The FDA staged a raid on the clinic at 9:00 A.M., kicking down the door. Six armed police officers, in flak jackets, with guns drawn accompanied the FDA agents. It was as if Barney Fife had gotten hold of a lot of federal funding. This show of force, no doubt, was in case the good doctor, in a fit of pique, threw a hypodermic at one of the officers.

Dr. Wright apparently brought on the raid by his dangerous practice of using injectable B-vitamins without preservatives. The FDA claims that it was Dr. Wright's criminal behavior, and not the fact that he was suing them for an earlier illegal seizure that led to the government's heavy-handed approach, which is usually reserved for loners living in Idaho, crack houses and Texas cults.

After the raid, the FDA regional director, a recent graduate of the "Barney Fife School of Criminal Investigations" displayed a vial of moldy magnesium to reporters. "This stuff can kill you!" the excited agent said with so much animation that the bullet fell out of his shirt pocket. Of course what he failed to tell the reporters was that the vial was procured from Dr. Wright's dumpster. So either it was garbage or Dr. Wright has the strangest product distribution system in Washington State.

The FDA in its campaign against Dr. Wright has found the funding for court time, even though no charges have been filed against him. It has expended manpower to go through the clinic's garbage, interview former employees and conduct an investigation that makes the OJ trial look like a minor traffic case. Considering that the U.S. government can't muster the resources to inspect more than 1% of the meat in this country, it's amazing what a bureaucracy can do when it really tries.

All of this effort is being expended to investigate a doctor with impeccable credentials by an agency that allows carcinogenic nitrites to be sold without a warning label, carcinogenic formaldehyde to be in building materials, and allows a wide variety of deadly additives to remain in our food supply. Drugs approved by the FDA are responsible for at least 1,182 deaths from 1983 to 1987, while no documented cases of death caused by vitamin supplements were reported in the same period.

You be the judge. Is the FDA protecting the public? Or does it have an ax to grind with physicians who practice natural health care?

Sorry, I had to get that off of my chest. Back to our lunch. Let's say that you have a typical iceberg lettuce salad. You use a commercial dressing; a low-fat one, since you're watching your weight. Here are the ingredients of a typical low-fat ranch dressing: Water; partially hydrogenated soybean oil; cultured nonfat buttermilk solids; sugar, modified food starch; salt; natural flavors; sodium caseinate; vinegar; phosphoric acid; onion (dehydrated); garlic (dehydrated); monosodium glutamate (enhances flavor [actually tricks your nervous system into thinking that it tastes good]); propylene glycol alginate; mono and diglycerides; sorbic acid; lactic acid; spice; artificial flavor;

xanthan gum; disodium inositate and disodium guanylate; parsley (dehydrated); calcium disodium EDTA; THBQ; and citric acid.

Here's a synopsis of the ingredients.

Water: The most plentiful ingredient in this product. This is a product that advertises itself to be 91% fat free. Since the manufacturer is talking about volume and not total calories, this can be accomplished by watering down the dressing. What's an easy way to make something that's 20% fat into something that's 10% fat? Double the volume by adding water.

Partially hydrogenated soybean oil: Hydrogenation turns an unsaturated fat into a saturated one. It changes the configuration of the fat molecule, creating something known as a trans fatty acid. On a molecular level, this is like turning a right-handed glove into a left-handed one. The result is something that can't really be used by the body. Trans fatty acids are actually worse than useless. They interfere with normal fat metabolism and have been linked to heart disease. They have a half-life in the body of 51 days. This means that it takes 51 days for your body to get rid of half of the trans fatty acids you eat. In other words, after 51 days, half of this hydrogenated oil is still in your system. In another 51 days you'll still have one-fourth of it. After another 51 days (153 days total) you'll still have one-eighth of the trans fatty acids in your system.

Cultured nonfat buttermilk solids: Probably better than illiterate nonfat buttermilk solids. Actually, it's much like powdered milk.

Modified food starch: This is starch that has been chemically altered to make it water soluble. Several different chemicals are used, such as propylene oxide, succinic anhydride, 1-octenyl succinic anhydride, aluminum sulfate and sodium hydroxide. You have no way of knowing what was used. In David Steinman's book *Diet for a Poisoned Planet*, he expresses concern about aluminum sulfate being used to modify food starch because there is a possible link between aluminum and Alzheimer's disease.

Natural flavors: Flavor from food that has had only minimal processing, without anything synthetic or any added chemical.

Sodium caseinate: This is the principle protein of cow's milk.

Vinegar: Finally, something you can recognize as a food that you would find in your own kitchen.

46

Phosphoric acid: This is an acid made from phosphate rock. The FDA considers it safe. Steinman makes the point that you can clean rust off of a chrome bumper with it.

Salt: Something else that is familiar. Since the connection between Alzheimer's disease and aluminum has been mentioned, you may want to read the label on your table salt. You'll notice that it contains aluminum (sodium silico aluminate) as an anticaking agent. Sea salt, kosher salt and pickling salt are all free of aluminum.

Onion and garlic: Good God! More food. This could get to be a habit.

Monosodium glutamate: Also known as MSG, which causes Chinese Restaurant Syndrome (chest pain, numbness and headache after eating). MSG causes brain damage in young rodents. Female animals treated with MSG had fewer pregnancies and smaller litters.

Propylene glycol alginate: Seaweed derivative. The FDA considers it safe.

Mono and diglycerides: Used as stabilizers and emulsifiers. According to Steinman, these can occur in nature, but are usually synthetically made. In his book, Steinman cites studies that show certain types of mono and diglycerides have caused decreased growth in mice, others have caused enlarged kidneys and decrease in the size of testes. (The poor mice probably were not sure whether they were coming or going.)

Sorbic acid: This is acetic acid. It is harmless.

Lactic acid: This occurs naturally in sour milk. The FDA considers it safe.

Spice: It now has sugar and spice (and everything nice?).

Artificial flavor: By definition, something not found in nature, although it may have components that are found in nature. Whatever it is, the manufacturer has opted not to tell you in detail what the substance is. It's sort of a mystery chemical.

Xanthan gum: Produced by fermentation of corn sugar. Xanthan gum thickens and helps the dressing to pour well. No known toxicity.

Disodium inositate: A flavor enhancer. No known toxicity.

Parsley: Another food.

Calcium disodium EDTA: Ethylenediaminetetraacetate. No kidding, my kids didn't just play with the keyboard. EDTA is used to bind materials that are undesirable in food. It hides metallic tastes and other undesirable flavors and colors in the food. This means that the dressing might taste a little weird without the EDTA (small wonder).

THBQ: Tertiarybutylhydroquinone. Food manufacturers had a hard time getting this approved, which means that even the FDA wasn't sure it should be on the market. Think about that. According to Ruth Winter's book, death has occurred from ingestion of five grams (about one-fifth of an ounce). Eating one gram can cause nausea, vomiting, ringing in the ears, delirium, a sense of suffocation and collapse. But hey, now the dressing can have a long shelf life.

Citric acid: One of the safer additives.

In a typical lunch of a sandwich and salad, here's a list of the harmful chemicals you consume: Mono and diglycerides (possible mutagens); benzoyl peroxide (irritant, acne medicine); potassium bromate (poison, possible carcinogen); calcium sulfate (plaster of Paris); ammonium chloride (safe, but one gram can cause vomiting and nausea); brominated vegetable oil (deadly poison, stored in the body); yellow #6 (possible link to kidney and adrenal tumors); red #40 (possible carcinogen); sodium nitrite (known carcinogen); partially hydrogenated oil (harms fat metabolism, linked to heart disease); aspartame (linked to brain cancer and other health problems); modified food starch (possibly harmful it aluminum was used, you have no way of knowing); EDTA (to help hide the weird taste of the other chemicals); THBQ (deadly poison), and a host of nonharmful chemicals. *Bon appetite!*

If this is a typical lunch for you, is it any wonder that you're tired? Is there any wonder why the cost of health care has skyrocketed? Are you still surprised that the average American consumes 10 pounds of chemical additives each year? Get yourself a copy of *A Consumer's Dictionary of Food Additives,* and take a walk through your supermarket reading labels. You'll be amazed at what you used to consume.

Let's consider an alternative lunch. We'll still have a sandwich. We'll even use a commercially available bread, whole wheat bread from the "Natural Ovens of Manitowoc, Wisconsin." Here's a list of ingredients of a loaf of their 100% whole grain bread: Stone ground whole wheat flour, flax seed, oat bran, wheat germ, barley malt, canola oil, yeast, sea salt and honey. We'll have a salad, since we're listening to the American Cancer Society. Our second salad will be made with spinach and the dressing will be plain olive oil (extra virgin) and vinegar. Instead of bologna, we will have turkey breast. Instead of a diet soft drink, we will have water. Our second lunch has no chemical additives.

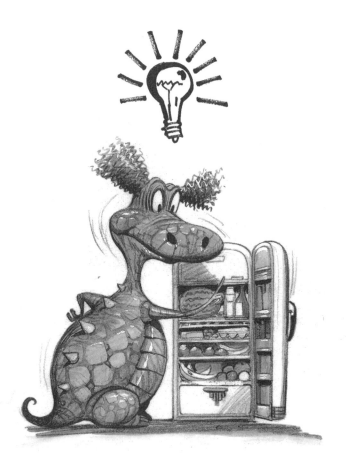

Even if chemicals were not a consideration in the first lunch, it still would not be as good as our second lunch. Compare the vitamin and mineral content of the two lunches.

A Tale of Two Sandwiches

Lunch #1—Bologna on white bread with a lettuce salad

Nutrient	Bread	Bologna	Lettuce	Total
Calories	128	214.2	15	357.2
Fat	1.8 g	16.1 g	0	17.9 g
Protein	4.0 g	14.0 g	1.0 g	19.0 g
Carbohydrate	23.0 g	2.14 g	2.0 g	27.14 g
Vitamin B1	0.11 mg	0.036 mg	0.05 mg	0.196 mg
Vitamin B2	0.14 mg	0.18 mg	0.05 mg	0.37 mg
Folic acid	0	0	55 mcg	55 mcg
Niacin	1.8 mg	3.9 mg	0	5.7 mg
Pantothenic acid	0.2 mg	0	0.05 mg	0.25 mg
Vitamin B6	0	0.18 mg	0.05 mg	0.23 mg
Vitamin B12	0	0.44 mcg	0	0.44 mcg
Sodium	52 mg	792 mg	10 mg	854 mg
Potassium	52 mg	189 mg	160 mg	401 mg
Calcium	60 mg	92.8 mg	20 mg	172.8 mg
Magnesium	10 mg	14.3 mg	10 mg	34.3 mg
Zinc	0.3 mg	2.3 mg	0.2 mg	2.8 mg
Phosphorus	52 mg	157 mg	20 mg	229 mg
Iron	1.36 mg	1.29 mg	0.5 mg	3.15 mg
Vitamin A (IU)	0	0	330 IU	330 IU
Vitamin E (IU)	0	0	0.35 IU	0.35 IU
Essential fatty acids	0	0	0	0
Vitamin C	0	0	5 mg	5 mg
Manganese	0	0	0.15 mg	0.15 mg

Lunch #2—Turkey on whole wheat with a spinach salad

Nutrient	Bread	Turkey	Spinach	Total
Calories	140	157	24	311
Fat	2 g	3.2 g	0	5.2 g
Protein	9 mg	29.9 mg	3.2 mg	42.1 g
Carbohydrate	33 mg	0	4 mg	37 g
Vitamin B1	0.35 mg	0.6 mg	0.1 mg	1.05 mg
Vitamin B2	0.17 mg	0.13 mg	0.2 mg	0.5 mg
Folic acid	80 mcg	6 mcg	220 mcg	306 mcg
Niacin	3.8 mg	6.8 mg	1.0 mg	11.6 mg
Pantothenic acid	0.2 mg	0.68 mg	0.1 mg	0.98 mg
Vitamin B6	0.88 mg	0.54 mg	0.24 mg	1.66 mg
Vitamin B12	0.45 mcg	0.37 mcg	0	0.82 mcg
Sodium	100 mg	63 mg	108 mg	271 mg
Potassium	200 mg	285 mg	624 mg	1109 mg
Calcium	160 mg	21 mg	112 mg	293 mg
Magnesium	35 mg	26 mg	88 mg	139 mg
Zinc	3.8 mg	2 mg	0.6 mg	6.4 mg
Phosphorus	160 mg	208 mg	56 mg	424 mg
Iron	0	1.4 mg	3.1 mg	4.5 mg
Vitamin A (IU)	0	0	7200 IU	7200 IU
Vitamin E (IU)	1 IU	0	2.7 IU	3.7 IU
Essential fatty acids	0	600 mg	0	600 mg
Vitamin C	0	0	32 mg	32mg
Manganese	0.6 mg	0.02 mg	1.0 mg	1.62 mg

Consider the nutritional differences between these two meals. Meal #2 has more than six times as much vitamin C as meal #1. It has 50% more riboflavin; seven times as much vitamin B6; five times as much B1; over 21 times as much vitamin A; 50% more calcium; about four times as much magnesium; twice as much niacin; almost 10 times as much vitamin E; two and a half times as much zinc; four times as much pantothenic acid; six times as much folic acid; twice as much vitamin B12 and over 10 times as much manganese. And meal #2 contains essential fatty acids, which aren't even present in the first meal.

The second meal is lacking in a few things provided by the first meal. Carcinogenic nitrites, THBQ, bromate and other dangerous additives are not present.

This comparison is just to show you the difference between two meals and to show you how important small changes in diet can be. Not getting vitamins in your meals and consuming chemical additives causes fatigue. Things in your diet, which you consume on a regular basis, may be undermining your health and making you tired.

This is just a simple and obvious comparison made between two meals that are available in any supermarket. The differences between the meals is important, because the lack of vitamins and minerals in meals like #1, and the burden of eating chemically laden food places on your liver, cause fatigue.

There is no need to worry about the issues of vegetarianism, organic produce, food combining whether or not dairy products should be consumed or other more sweeping changes you could make to your diet—if you are still consuming food that is full of additives and devoid of vitamins, like the food in the first lunch. You don't need to become some sort of fanatic. It may seem to you that the world is divided into two camps. One camp has the health "nuts": people wearing Berkenstocks and prints, driving Volvos and lecturing you about this additive and that chemical. They always seem to be eating some amorphous congealed mass, purchased in a health food store and tasting like something you once smelled on a farm. The other camp is the "screw it, I'm going to die anyway" crowd, stuffing their faces with Coke and Cheetos. Don't feel pressured, and don't feel that you have to go off the deep end and start eating things that smell like a farm animal had it first. Just begin to make healthy decisions. You can eat normal food, just wean yourself from packaged and processed foods.

You do not have to disrupt your lifestyle to eat better. You can still enjoy a meal of a sandwich and a salad, but what a world of difference if you take a little time and pay attention to the quality of your food. Increasing the amount of nutrients and decreasing the sugar and added chemicals you get in your food will improve your health. Get the most food value out of each meal you eat and you will have incredible energy. Increasing the amount of nutrients and decreasing the sugar and added chemicals will improve your health.

Chemicals and additives drain your energy. The constant chemical bombarding you get with additives, chemicals and pesticides causes fatigue and can eventually lead to allergies and immune system problems. Considering the fact that everything that takes place in your body involves chemical reactions, it should be obvious that introducing chemicals on your body that do not belong there can have far-reaching implications on your health and energy. Denying the body vitamins and minerals by eating food that is nutrient deficient undermines health. In order to survive, the body must conserve energy. It becomes fatigued.

Patients who eat nutrient deficient, additive and sugar-loaded diets are continually asking questions like, "Doc, do you think that taking bee pollen will give me more energy?" It's how we're trained to think of health care: I can do anything to my body that I want to as long as I find the right pill to make me feel better. Unfortunately, that is a poor strategy for maintaining your health and energy.

If you are fatigued, the very first place you need to look is in your diet. This is like checking for gas if your car doesn't start. It is basic. No exotic herb, no medical regimen, not even extract from humming bird testicles will work if you do not have good nutrition.

Go on a caveman diet. This doesn't mean that you have to eat brontosaurus steaks and pterodactyl eggs. You don't have to go to the snack bar at Jurassic Park. Simply eat foods that were available 10,000 years ago. If the food comes in a bottle, box or a can, avoid it. Stop eating refined foods and those with chemical additives. Drink plenty of water. Get plenty of rest.

If your car doesn't function, you look at the simple, basic things— the battery, gas, whether or not it is in drive—before you pull out the engine and have it overhauled. This the way it should be with your body. Good nutrition is not an alternative therapy, like many doctors would have you believe. It is a fundamental part of good health.

Good nutrition is especially important considering the changes in agriculture over the past 100 years. The use of chemical fertilizers depletes the soil of trace nutrients like zinc, molybdenum, manganese and other minerals. A vegetable will not contain anything that is not in the soil that it grows in. Chemical fertilizers enable farmers to grow large, attractive produce that has very little food value. Who hasn't taken a bite out of a nice, big, bright red apple only to find that it tastes like Styrofoam?

One hundred years ago, fewer than 3% of all deaths were from cancer. Today, one in four American men and one in five American women die of cancer. According to the National Cancer Institute, between 1950 and 1985 cancer in children increased 32%; bladder cancer increased 51%; testicular cancer increased 81%; kidney and renal pelvis cancer increased 82%; and non-Hodgkin's lymphoma (linked with pesticide exposure) increased by 123%. Much of this increase in cancer can be attributed to food additives and pesticides, and is compounded by the fact that much of our food is depleted of vitamins.

As more of the population becomes aware of the danger of chemicals, it is becoming increasingly popular to buy pesticide-free, organic produce. Two grocery chains, Whole Foods and Fresh Fields, have been opening stores around the country. They sell additive-free food and have selections of organically grown produce.

If you do not have enough energy, it is important to pay attention to the quality of your food. You need to eat whole foods that are high in nutrition. You need to avoid additives and other chemicals as much as possible.

Chemicals cause fatigue. If you have ever had a hangover, you know the effect chemicals can have on you. A hangover is simply a state of chemical toxicity. Your fatigue may be due to a chemical "hangover."

Fat

In the midst of the chemical onslaught your body goes through, the chief dietary villain the media and the medical profession have chosen is fat. People are eating turkey bologna and salami, loaded with cancer-causing nitrites, with a secure feeling that they are eating properly. Such products advertise that they are low in fat, and people who eat them sincerely believe that they are eating healthily.

Other products that advertise being low-fat are loaded with chemicals. Consider the low-fat dressing a few pages back. Low-fat doesn't automatically mean healthy. Actually the word lite is an ancient Sanskrit word meaning: "full of chemicals."

The food pyramid, designed to replace the now-defunct four food groups, makes no distinction between refined and whole grains. People are being taught that grain products are low in fat and good for them. As a result, they are consuming tons of white, refined noodles, breads and other nutrient-deficient, chemically laden products, thinking that they are eating healthily.

Fat is not the unmixed evil that many experts would have you believe. In fact, many people who suffer from fatigue are on low-fat diets.

If your fat consumption is too low, you will not absorb oil-soluble nutrients very well. You become deficient in essential fatty acids, vitamin A, vitamin E, vitamin K and possibly vitamin D (although vitamin D is a popular food additive and not many people are lacking in it.) Fat is necessary for the proper functioning of the endocrine system. Cholesterol is necessary for production of adrenal hormones.

Deficiencies in oil-soluble nutrients can affect the skin, the musculoskeletal system, the endocrine system and the immune system. If your diet is too low in fat, you may experience fatigue, dry skin, frequent colds, frequent bladder infections, menstrual problems, allergies, muscle fatigability and even tension headaches.

Dr. Pritikin, and more recently, Dr. Dean Ornish, have had success with heart patients by putting them on a 10% fat diet. Their success has many erroneously believing that everyone needs to be on a 10% fat diet. Actually, a diet this low in fat is a medical treatment meant to be used in extreme cases. It is, in itself, an extreme measure.

Many people do well on low-fat diets because the worst foods in their diets are fats. Animals are at the top of the food chain. Insecticides permeate everything in the environment, including water and vegetation. Animals consume water and vegetation and store the chemicals in their fat. Over time, the chemicals in the animals' tissue become more concentrated.

Butter and cheese are very high in pesticide residues. The FDA tested cheddar cheese from around the nation and found 100 pesticide and industrial chemical residues in the samples. These included BHC, DDT, dieldrin, heptachlor, HCB and octachlor, which were found in 25% of the samples.

Fatty foods potentiate carcinogenic effects of the chemicals in the food. In other words, if you consume chemicals in the presence of fat, the chemicals are more dangerous.

Less than 1% of all meat is tested for carcinogens. In 1988 an internal audit by the inspector general's office of the USDA discovered that the tainted meat had been sold for consumption, even after federal inspectors found that it was chemically contaminated.

Meat and dairy products not only have chemicals from the environment, they have chemicals that are purposely given to the animals by the farmers. Half of all the antibiotics sold in this country are purchased by farmers. They are added to animal feed, indiscriminately, at the discretion of the farmer.

Dairy cows are now being given bovine growth hormone, or BGH. The manufacturer prefers it to be called bovine somatotrophin (Bovine somatotrophin is a less-threatening name. This is better marketing. Of course that would make the acronym BS, which probably is more appropriate.) The FDA has given farmers permission to use BGH without having to tell consumers.

The FDA justifies this lack of consumer information by telling the public that BGH isn't found in the milk. Of course, nothing is said about BGH undermining the animals' health, making it necessary for the farmer to give more antibiotics and other drugs that will find their way into the milk. Even if BGH were totally harmless, as the FDA claims, there has been enough outcry from consumers to justify labeling.

In general, there is always the possibility that meat and dairy products contain chemicals. A lot of the problem has to do with how the animals are raised. Hog barns are built with slatted floors, over large pits where the excrement is collected below. The hogs are in tiny stalls and inhale the fumes of their own waste, 24 hours a day. The hogs are never allowed outside. Because of the crowded, filthy conditions, pneumonia is always a threat.

In order to prevent pneumonia, drugs are given to the hogs. Sulfa drugs are very popular among hog farmers because they are cheap. One of the more popular drugs is sulfanethazine, which has been linked to thyroid problems in humans and is a possible carcinogen. Ten percent of the slaughtered hogs tested (remember that only 1% of all animals are tested), have sulfamethazine residues. Sulfamethazine is only one chemical. Animal fat has a lot of chemicals in it. It is wise to reduce your consumption of it.

Not all fat is created equal. It is important for you to understand the difference between fats. Vegetable oils, raw nuts and avocados are sources of good fat and should not be completely shunned. Some kinds of fat should be avoided, but not all. If you are careful about the quality of the fat you eat, you can eat a diet that is 20 or even 30% fat. Some sources of fat follow:

58

Meat and dairy: High in saturated fat and high in chemicals. There is wisdom in eating poultry and fish, which are low in fat, and selecting low-fat cuts of meat. You can buy organically grown meat, free range chickens and dairy products from cows that have not been given antibiotics. If you eat animal products, it is wise to find animals that have not been fed steroids or antibiotics, and animals that have not been raised on factory-farms that abuse them and put out an unhealthy product.

Vegetable oils: At the turn of the century, all salad oil was produced by pressing flax seeds. This oil was very high in essential fatty acids. Now most oils are extracted with heat or chemicals. Once an oil has been heated, it has absolutely no nutritional value. It may even be toxic. You should stay away from oils that have been heat or chemically extracted and buy only cold-pressed oils. If the oil is in a clear bottle, exposed to light, you should not consume it. The naturally obtained oils are not stored this way because they can become rancid. If the oil is in a clear bottle, exposed to light, it probably was extracted with heat or chemicals.

Heat damages oil and potentially makes it carcinogenic. This is why you should never eat deep-fried foods. It's okay to sauté foods in olive oil. Never reheat or reuse oil.

Olive oil is relatively stable to heat. You can sauté food in olive oil and not worry too much about it being toxic. There are different grades of olive oil. The highest quality imported olive oil is graded as extra virgin. The next highest quality is virgin, which is between 1.0 and 3.3 percent acid. Olive oil which has been graded as pure is the lowest grade of olive oil, because the producers thought it would be better than grading it as crappy, which would be bad for sales. It's the same reason you can't buy a "small" soda pop or popcorn at the movies. Olive oil grades are a lot like going to the snack bar at the movies and the soda pop comes in three sizes: large, extra large and jumbo. Pure olive oil has a high acid content that has been neutralized with chemicals; it is not of acceptable quality. Domestic olive oil has three grades: virgin—the first pressing and highest American grade of olive oil; refined—second pressing which has added chemicals to neutralize the acidity; and refined olive residue oil—good for crankcases or to substitute at a "Wesson" party. When buying olive oil, look for the words *virgin* or *extra virgin* on the label.

Hydrogenated or partially hydrogenated oil: Avoid these like the plague. They are implicated in heart disease. They interfere with normal fat metabolism. They stay in the body for a very long time. Hydrogenation is a way of artificially saturating an unsaturated fat. This makes an oil into a solid and makes it ship and store better. Margarine and mayonnaise are made with hydrogenated oils. Hydrogenated and partially hydrogenated oils are found in a lot of packaged and convenience foods.

Avocados and nuts: These are excellent sources of oil-soluble nutrients. Make sure that the nuts are raw; do not eat roasted nuts. Peanut butter, cashew butter, almond butter and tahinni are very nutritious, but get the organic version. Smooth commercial peanut butters have added sugar, hydrogenated oil and other chemicals. Buy peanut butter which has the oil separate from the rest of the peanut butter, like Smuckers and Holsum. If you read the label of these products, you will see that they only have peanuts and salt.

Fried foods: Carcinogenic empty calories. Avoid them. A diet too high in fat can make it difficult to lose weight. Just make sure that you eat fat, even good fats, in moderation.

Vegetarianism

It is not necessary to become a vegetarian to become thin and healthy. There are, however, some health advantages to vegetarian eating. Vegetarians usually have less fat and fewer chemicals in their diet. The vegetarian diet is easier to digest than a diet that contains meat and dairy. As a rule, vegetarian meals are usually much lower in calories than meals containing animal products.

While it is not absolutely necessary that you become a vegetarian, it would be helpful if you changed how you think about food. Most Americans don't think a meal is complete without meat. In many other cultures beans and bread is a meal. In this country they are an appetizer, snack or side dish.

Vegetarians often suffer from fatigue, especially salad bar vegetarians who live on iceberg lettuce and bread. Many vegetarians eat a lot of refined food. Nutrient deficiency is a problem for many of them. It's not that the vegetarian diet is inherently low in certain nutrients; it's just that people who eat meat get certain vitamins easier than vegetarians do.

Many vegetarians are deficient in vitamin B12, which is a

nutrient that is in meat and dairy products. Vegetarians can get it from their intestinal bacteria, but good bowel health is necessary for this. If a vegetarian's bowel is not healthy, he or she may be deficient in B12. A deficiency in B12 can cause fatigue among other things, and supplementation may necessary for many vegetarians.

Many argue that the vegetarians tend to be protein deficient because the protein available to them is not as complete as animal protein. A complete protein is one that contains all eight essential amino acids. An essential amino acid is one that the body cannot manufacture; it has to be gotten from the diet. Animal proteins tend to have all eight essential amino acids. Most vegetables do not have complete proteins. They may have some of the essential amino acids, but not all of them. A vegetarian usually has to eat more than one food to get a complete protein. If you eat a whole grain and a legume (bean, pea or nut), you get the same quality protein as a steak. Quinoa, a grain, is also a complete protein.

Many people become vegetarians because they don't digest meat well or because eating meat doesn't make them feel very good. This is often due to the stomach not producing enough hydrochloric acid. These people tend to live on starch and leafy vegetables, because these foods are easy to digest. Fatigue, due to a deficiency of essential amino acids, vitamin B12 and many minerals, is often a problem. Supplementation may be necessary. Taking vitamin B12 as a nasal gel, a multimineral and an amino acid supplement (containing all eight of the essential amino acids) often gives these people incredible energy.

Vitamin B12 deficiency is a common source of fatigue in vegetarians. Many times the deficiency is due to a problem absorbing the vitamin. It is better to take B12 as a nasal gel or a sublingual spray than in a pill form.

If you are not a vegetarian, try some vegetarian meals. Get out of the habit of eating animal products with every meal. You will find eating vegetarian meals very satisfying. The meals are lower in chemicals than meals containing meat and dairy. These meals are also easier to digest and will not weigh you down the way meat and dairy do. Here are some recipes to get you started.

Baba Ghanoush

3 large eggplants	3 cloves of garlic, crushed
1/4 cup tahinni	juice of 3 lemons

Broil the eggplants until the skin blisters. Peel off the skin or rub it off under cold tap water. Squeeze out as much of the bitter juice as possible and remove the seeds. The idea is to use the white pulpy part of the eggplant. Place the eggplant in a food processor, add the tahinni, lemon juice and garlic (crushed in a garlic press). Blend everything into a fine puree. Salt to taste. Eat it with whole wheat pita bread, have a salad or cut up vegetables on the side. Can also be used as a bread spread, like hommus.

Hommus

1 cup chickpeas	juice of 2 lemons
2 cloves of garlic	1/4 cup of tahinni

Soak the chickpeas overnight and boil them until tender, about an hour (or you can cheat and use canned chick peas). Place them in a food processor, add the tahinni, lemon juice and the garlic (crushed in a garlic press). Blend everything into a fine puree. Serve as a dip with whole wheat pita bread, add some cut up vegetables or a salad and it makes a meal. This is a very tasty dish. It can be eaten as a meal or can be used as a spread instead of butter.

Vegetables and Rice

2 cups cooked brown rice

1 finely chopped sweet
red pepper

1/2 small onion,
chopped

1 stalk celery,
sliced with leaves

1/2 cup water

2 tablespoons fresh dill

salt and pepper to taste

1/2 cup chopped parsley

1 cup fresh green beans (cut, 1" long)

2 medium zucchini, sliced
and quartered

1 tablespoon lemon juice

3 tablespoons butter

1/4 cup white wine

Combine rice and parsley, arrange as a bed on a large serving platter.
Cook zucchini and beans in water, until tender and drain.
Sauté onion, pepper and celery in butter with dill, lemon and pepper.
Add wine. Add this mixture to the other vegetables. Place the mixture
on the rice. Serve.

Zucchini and Tomato

2 medium zucchini, sliced
and quartered

1 large sweet onion
(like walla walla), diced

1/2 cup tomato sauce

1/4 cup fresh oregano leaves

2 large tomatoes, cut into wedges

1/4 cup rice vinegar

1 clove garlic, crushed

1/4 cup fresh basil leaves

Combine all of the ingredients in a small saucepan, cover it and heat on
a very small flame until the vegetables are tender (about 30 minutes).
Serve it over brown rice.

Veggie Burgers

1/3 cup finely chopped sweet red pepper	1/3 cup finely chopped celery
1/3 cup finely chopped carrots	2 tbs. finely chopped onions
6 black olives, finely chopped	1 tbs. finely chopped parsley
1 egg beaten	1 tbs. olive oil
1/4 cup tomato sauce	1 cup ground, raw, sunflower seeds
3 tbs. wheat germ	salt and pepper to taste

Mix all of the ingredients thoroughly in a bowl. Make into four patties and place them in a greased baking dish. Bake at 350 degrees for 15 minutes (until brown). Turn patties over and bake another 15 minutes (until brown). Serve as a sandwich, using whole grain bread.

64

Carrot and Zucchini Stir Fry

1 cup carrots, cut julienne style	1 cup zucchini, cut julienne style
1 tsp. sesame oil	1 tbs. peanut oil
1 clove garlic, crushed	1 tbs. fresh, grated ginger

Heat peanut and sesame oil with the garlic and ginger. When oil is hot, add carrots and zucchini. Mix while cooking for 2-3 minutes, until vegetables are tender, but still a little crunchy. Serve over brown rice.

Ratatouille

1 eggplant	2 zucchini
2 sweet red peppers	3 small onions
(or green peppers)	
6 cloves of garlic	1 cup of tomatoes
1 cup chicken broth	1/4 cup chopped, fresh basil
salt and pepper to taste	

Peel eggplant and cut into 1 inch cubes. Slice zucchini. Coarsely dice tomatoes, onions and peppers. Peel and crush the garlic. Steam the vegetables until tender. Heat the chicken broth and simmer the vegetables and garlic in it for three minutes. Top with basil, salt and pepper.

Creole Pinto Beans

1/2 pound of dried	1 tbs. olive oil
pinto beans	
1 medium onion, chopped	1 green pepper, chopped
1 stalk of celery, chopped	2 cups tomatoes, chopped
1/4 tsp. dried thyme	1/2 tsp. cayenne pepper
1/2 tsp. black pepper	1 clove of garlic, minced
1/2 tsp. sweet paprika	1/2 tsp. sea salt
2 tbs. tomato paste	

Boil the pinto beans for 20-30 minutes, let stand while preparing the other ingredients. Heat oil and sauté onion and green pepper for two minutes. Add celery and tomatoes and sauté until all of the vegetables are tender. Add tomato paste and all of the spices. Simmer for about 15 minutes. Add beans. If mixture is too dry, add a little water. Good over brown rice or whole wheat pasta. For what it's worth, you can use any bean you like if you prefer not to have pinto beans. The dish is easier to make if you substitute canned pinto or canned kidney beans.

Stress

Hans Selye conducted some experiments which today may have gotten animal rights activists upset (or at least gotten him a visit from the Soys in the Hood). Selye's assistant, Gunter, is credited with much of Hans' success by exercising a little damage control. Gunter wisely convinced Hans to use rats for his experiments, instead of Selye's first choice, baby seals, and saved the project from being beset upon by militant vegetarians.

Thanks to Gunter, Selye conducted his experiments on rats, which hardly raised an eyebrow. Of course it was the 1930s and this sort of thing was not as big of an issue as it is today. Also, no one seems to care if you experiment on an ugly animal.

The experiments involved creating stress in rats. Hans' early attempts at subjecting them to IRS audits were not very successful. Being a lab rat doesn't pay very well, and most of the animals were using the short form. Gunter again suggested some changes and saved the experiment. The rats were made to tread water with their legs tied until they became exhausted and died. Many humans would find this less stressful than an IRS audit, but it worked very well with the rats.

Dr. Selye took the rats at various stages of their ordeal and dissected out their adrenal glands. He found that the adrenal glands responded to stress in three distinct stages. In the initial stage, the adrenal glands enlarge and the blood supply to them increases. As the stress continues, the adrenal glands begin to shrink. Eventually, if the stress continues, the adrenal glands reach the third stage, which is adrenal exhaustion.

You may ask yourself, "What do rat adrenal glands have to do with me?" You may even be saying to yourself, "That's disgusting, what he did to the rats. How do I join the Soys in the 'Hood?" You may be thinking, "What's an adrenal gland?" You may even be thinking, "I'm tired. I think that I'll read this later."

If you are tired, it may well have to do with your adrenal glands. The adrenal glands produce their hormones in response to stress. They are responsible for the fight or flight response. In a stressful situation, they make your blood pressure increase, transfer blood from your intestines to your extremities, increase your heart rate, suppress your immune system and increase your blood's clotting ability.

This response is meant to be short-lived. When primitive man walked through the forest, he'd see a saber tooth tiger, which would really freak him out since saber tooth tigers were supposed to have been extinct for thousands of years. His heart rate would increase; his pupils would dilate; his blood would go out of his digestive system and into his arms and legs; his blood clotting ability would improve; he would become more aware and his blood pressure would rise. At that point he'd either pick up a stick and try to fight the animal or run like hell to go find a veterinary orthodontist. The physiological changes brought on by the adrenal glands would make the body more efficient at doing either of those things. It is called the fight or flight response.

If he survived the ordeal, chances are it would be a while before such a strain was put on the adrenal glands and the rest of his body. He would have an opportunity to relax, eat nuts and berries, and a little saber tooth tiger steak, if he was lucky. His adrenal glands would have a chance to recover.

Many people in modern society do not have the luxury of a recovery period for their overworked adrenal glands. The changes caused by the overproduction of adrenal hormones stay with them. The stimulation of the adrenal glands causes a decrease in the immune system function, so an individual under constant stress will tend to catch colds and have other immune system problems, including allergies. Blood flow to the digestive tract is decreased. **Stress causes many digestive problems** such as indigestion, colitis and irritable bowel. Adrenal hormones cause an increase in the blood clotting ability, so prolonged stress can lead to arterial plaquing and heart disease.

Worrying makes your adrenal glands work. Relaxing and thinking peaceful thoughts enables them to rest and heal. That is why yoga and meditation are so good for you. You go a long way in preserving your health and energy if you do not fret about things over which you have no control. It's the amount of worry and not necessarily the size of the problem that stresses your adrenal glands. If you worry a lot about little problems, you get to do as much damage to your adrenal glands as someone who really has a lot of stress. If you can control your worrying when under stress, you minimize the damage stress does to your health. A wise man once said that worry is interest paid in advance on money you haven't even borrowed yet.

Selye described the progression of stress on the adrenal glands as the general adaptation syndrome. The first stage is called the alarm reaction. This is when someone (with healthy adrenal glands) can perform amazingly well when the need arises. The primitive man, seeing the saber tooth tiger, was able to run faster than he ever dreamed possible during the alarm reaction. If the stress continues, the body moves into the resistance stage, during which the adrenals become enlarged. The individual is responding to the stress and handling it. He or she may feel keyed up. The person may have cold, clammy hands, rapid pulse or reduced appetite, but hasn't begun to feel any of the more serious symptoms of the next stage, During the exhaustion stage the adrenals begin to fail to meet the demands placed upon them. During this stage, the individual begins to have a variety of symptoms including fatigue, digestive problems, obesity, depression, dizziness, fainting, allergies and many other problems.

Traditional medicine does not recognize functional hypoadrenia as a health problem. The only adrenal problem recognized by medicine is

Addison's disease, which is complete adrenal failure. This is pretty amazing since medicine recognizes that the thyroid can function at various levels, including borderline hypothryoid. Traditional medicine has taken the view that the adrenals are either working or they are not.

Functional hypoadrenia is recognized by many physicians who deal in natural health care. One thing these doctors look for in a patient with this problem is postural hypotension. This is when the patient's blood pressure drops when he or she stands up from a reclining position. Frequently the patient feels dizzy when getting up suddenly. There are other causes for such dizziness, such as blood pressure medication, hypoglycemia and central nervous system problems. Don't diagnose yourself. Get a physical examination.

Another thing the physician may look for is a rebound pupil. Normally when a light is shined into the eye, the pupil tightly constricts. In a person suffering from functional hypoadrenia, the pupil will constrict and dilate again, sometimes oscillating. This is why strong light frequently bothers such a patient.

People with weak adrenal glands frequently crave coffee and sugar, as well as salt. Sugar and caffeine stimulate the adrenal glands. It's as if your adrenal glands are two horses towing a wagon load of bricks up a mountain. Sugar or caffeine is the whip you use to get the horses to keep trying. What they need to get to the top of the mountain is nourishment and a rest period.

In order to effectively treat functional hypoadrenia, you must eliminate as much stress from your life as possible. Emotional stress is the kind of stress most people think of when stress is mentioned, but there are many different kinds of stress. There is thermal stress from being exposed to extremes of temperature. There is physical stress, from heavy physical work, poor posture, structural misalignments, lack of sleep and being overweight. There is chemical stress from ingesting food additives, exposure to pollutants and consumption of sugar and alcohol. Changes in blood sugar are also a form of chemical stress. Eating frequent, small meals is often very helpful, since people suffering from hypoadrenia are often hypoglycemic.

Situations are not always controllable, but stress is. Stress is cumulative. Emotional stress, structural stress and chemical stress all affect the body the same way. Your adrenal glands do not know the difference between an IRS audit, treading water or excessive sugar consumption. And excess sugar consumption will add to the stress of the IRS audit.

If you **reduce the stress that you can control,** stressful situations will not have as much of a physical effect on you. For instance, eating frequent meals and avoiding sugar will reduce stress on the adrenal glands. So even if you can't do anything about Aunt Millie and Uncle Edgar coming to spend the summer, you can reduce your stress by controlling your diet. Also, how you think of the stress will make a difference in the health of your adrenal glands. Aunt Millie's handy tips on how you should raise your kids or clean your house, or Uncle Edgar's penchant for eating everything that isn't nailed down (without offering to pay for groceries) won't make you crazy if you don't focus on it.

If there is a situation in your life that you can't control, reduce the stress in the areas of your life that you do control. Also, try to focus on the positive areas of your life and not on the one or two things that really stress you out. If your job or your relationship situation is not exactly perfect, or not completely under your control, you can still reduce the effect stress has on your body and adrenal glands by reducing other forms of stress that you can control and by controlling what you focus your mind on.

If you can't change your work situation, then improve your diet and get plenty of rest. Change how you think about your job situation. Focus on the positive: You do have a job, and you do eat regular meals. (Much of the world doesn't.) Just do the best you can and think of the things you can't control in positive terms. Jesus says in Luke 12:25, "And which of you with taking thought can add to his stature one cubit?" Or, to quote my teacher and spiritual advisor, Yogi Babaganoush, "Chill out man." Think to yourself, "What could be good about this situation?" Then take a minute to really look for positive answers.

Hanging on to anxiety over past situations is stressful. **Thought has power.** Worry gives you all of the physiologic responses of Selye's rats or the caveman facing the saber tooth tiger. It's a waste of energy and it undermines your health.

Your adrenal glands simply don't know the difference between imagined danger and real danger. This is why meditation and biofeedback have been so valuable in controlling stress. Doctors are beginning to find that laughter helps the prognosis of cancer patients. They even have patients watch sitcoms in the hospital: "Mr. Smith, it's time for your chemotherapy and 'Lucy' reruns."

Minimizing chemical stress is also important. There is plenty of chemical stress today. Environmental pollution, food additives, sugar, alcohol and caffeine contribute stress to your adrenal glands. You must remove chemical stresses from your diet—effortlessly and without putting yourself under pressure. Gradually improve your diet by removing chemical additives. Move toward a more organic way of eating. Enjoy the change without fretting over how your diet isn't perfect yet.

Ironically, stress often makes you crave the foods that are bad for you. While under stress, it's hard to be diligent in keeping additives out of the diet. Patients often complain that they have no time and can't eat properly. Lack of time really isn't the problem because raw nuts, fruits and vegetables do not have to be cooked and take no time to prepare. If it was sex, and not food preparation, you'd find the time. Lack of time is usually used as an excuse to give in to craving the wrong foods. Once you understand that, you can eat healthily with little effort. Do the habit control exercise at the end of the book. There is also a habit control exercise, as well as a stress reduction exercise available in the tape set that is designed to accompany this book.

Eating sugar and skipping meals are two things that are especially stressful to the adrenal glands. Your adrenals work to keep your blood sugar level. Eating sugar causes a temporary increase in blood sugar, which soon drops. Skipping meals also causes the blood sugar to drop. The adrenals then have to work to increase the blood sugar. Hypoadrena and hypoglycemia (low blood sugar) usually exist together.

There are other things you can do to treat the adrenal glands. In applied kinesiology, there are several reflex points that will improve adrenal function when manually stimulated. Chiropractic adjustments, massage and other types of bodywork reduce stress. Vitamin supplements, such as vitamin C, vitamin B complex and other nutrients are often helpful.

The stress reduction exercise at the end of the book will help you to reduce the stress you feel. The tape set that accompanies this book also contains the exercise.

One form of treatment, which is rather controversial, is the use of glandular supplements. Many practitioners frequently give their patients a supplement made from the adrenal glands of a cow or a sheep (with the active hormone removed). There is some evidence to support the value of these supplements. Radioactively labeled adrenal glandular substance has been found to go to the adrenal glands of the individual injected with the substance.

One of the problems with some brands of glandulars is inconsistency in the potency and the quality of the supplements. It may even be possible, that in some brands, not all of the hormone is removed. If the hormone is not completely removed from the gland, it works like a drug and can create problems.

Clinically, when a glandular substance is given to the patient who needs it, the results are often dramatic. Frequently, patients suffering from adrenal insufficiency improve when they take an adrenal glandular. They sometimes improve when given a glandular made of thymus. Frequently the thymus improves the immune system of someone suffering from allergies.

The intention here is not to get everyone to run out and take glandular substances. In fact, they can be harmful in some patients. This is only to inform you of some of the treatments available and that this is a subject that warrants further investigation. It would be interesting to see more research done on glandular substances. Usually glandulars are helpful to a patient in the exhaustion stage, but may overstimulate the glands if the patient is in one of the earlier stages. If this is something that you think you may want to try, get help from a physician who understands it. The issue of supplement quality alone makes it necessary to get professional expertise.

Some herbs, like ephedra and ma-huang stimulate the adrenals. Be careful with products like this; the herb stimulates the adrenals, it doesn't heal them or strengthen them. You initially feel great, but the herb will eventually push the adrenals into exhaustion. Once again, don't treat yourself. You may end up like the unfortunate Mr. Needlebrain.

You can improve your adrenal function without stressing the glands. The following steps will improve your health and help you to overcome the effects of stress.

Stress reduction: The exercise included at the end of the book will do a great deal to help ease your stress. Listening to the stress reduction tape is even more effective. Listen to it as often as you feel the need to. You can also meditate or do yoga. Avoid negative thinking. Exercise regularly. Make any changes in your life that reduce stress.

Avoid foods that are stressors: Avoid chemical additives, sugar, refined carbohydrates, caffeine, nicotine and alcohol.

Eat plenty of fresh vegetables and whole grains.

Snack frequently: Try not to go more than 2-3 hours without eating something.

Take a good quality vitamin B complex.

Structural Stress

Poor posture, bad ergonomics and tight muscles can be stressful and drain your energy. A muscle that is in spasm uses the same amount of energy as a muscle doing work. Your body doesn't know the difference between physical work and having a muscle spasm. Those tight upper back muscles at the end of a day's work are the equivalent of lifting something over and over again; the muscle uses energy and produces waste. It's doing work, but it's not accomplishing anything but making you tired and uncomfortable. It can be a major cause of fatigue.

Poor posture can affect your breathing, muscle tone and ultimately your energy level. Holding your head forward makes the muscles in your upper back and neck work very hard. It can cause muscle spasm. Poor posture also causes you to breathe shallowly, reducing the amount of oxygen reaching the tissues and reducing the flow of the lymphatic system. You have already seen the connection between shallow breathing and fatigue.

Good posture when viewed from the front consists of having you head balanced over your pelvis, hips level, shoulders level and head level. If you look at your body from the side, the ears should be directly above the shoulders and hip joints. The ear, shoulder and hip joint should form a line that is perpendicular to the ground. The spine should be straight, allowing only for the normal curves of the spine, the lumbar and cervical lordosis and the thoracic kyphosis.

Ergonomics literally means "laws of work" in Latin. It is the rules for posture, designing workstations, lifting and using proper body mechanics. In a job that is sedentary, involves staying in one position for a long time, or has repetitive motion, it is best to minimize the stress on the body. That is the purpose of ergonomics.

If you sit, the chair should support your lumbar spine, and have arm rests. The height of the chair should be adjustable to enable your feet to be level on the ground and your thighs level. Also, the chair should have wheels on it so you can get to other areas of your workstation without reaching. You should not have to reach higher than your shoulders or lower than your hips. If something is above your shoulders, use a step stool to reach it. Things that you use frequently should be in easy reach and you should not spend the day bending down or reaching up.

Working on a computer presents some unique ergonomics problems. Using proper ergonomics will help to make sure that you don't come down with "floppy disk" or other structural problems. Carpal tunnel syndrome is common in people who work on computers all day. Resting your wrists on a foam pad that sits at the base of your keyboard will help prevent carpal tunnel.

People working with computers tend to hold their head motionless for long periods of time. This is hard on your neck and upper back. Make absolutely sure that the screen is at eye level and that you don't hold your head forward, or look up or down for long periods of time. When working on a computer, do not go more than 10 minutes without moving your neck and shoulders. Set a timer, and every 10 minutes stretch and rotate your neck. This will reduce fatigue and spasm in the neck and upper back.

It is helpful if your monitor is capable of moving. There are monitor holders that pivot and extend like a desk lamp. Changing the monitor position throughout the day will help to reduce the strain on your neck and upper back.

One of the absolutely worse things you can do while working on a computer is to sit for long periods of time, motionless, with your head turned. People doing word processing and copying documents frequently sit this way. It is a common source of neck pain.

People who make their living talking on the telephone often suffer from neck pain and spasm. Many are in the habit of holding the receiver between their ear and shoulder. That is just asking for pain and muscle spasm. Use a headset if you spend a lot of time on the telephone.

Try this exercise: Let your head (but only your head) hang as far forward as is comfortable. With your fingertips, press firmly just below the base of the skull. Using a comfortable pressure, make tiny circles from the center out to your ears and back again. The exercise is from a booklet entitled *De-stress in 10 Minutes (Or Less)*. It's available from L.J. Hake and Associates. They do self-massage and relaxation workshops for people in stressful or sedentary jobs. The above exercise is just a sample from the booklet they use to teach the class. L.J. Hake and Associates, P.O. Box 417153, Chicago, IL 60641.

If you stand and work at a counter, it should be at a proper height so that you can work without bending. If you stand for long periods of time, it helps to put your foot on a small footrest about six inches in height. Change which foot is on the footrest from time to time.

Lifting should be done without bending at the waist. Bend your knees to get close to what you are lifting. Keep your back straight and bring the item in as close to your body as you can get it. Lift even small objects properly. The combination of bending at the waist and twisting the spine is very stressful and can cause you to injure your low back.

Even lifting something small off of the floor will cause a severe back injury if the person bends at the waist and twists to one side while bending. How often have you heard someone say, "I just picked up my pen (or the cap off the toothpaste, a nickel or my false teeth), and I got the worst pain in my back."

Ninety-eight percent of all Americans will have back pain at some point in their lives. There are specific back exercises that will help prevent back injury. If you are a sedentary individual, light exercise will generally help your posture, breathing and muscle tone. Structural stress can be handled in several ways. Stretching, exercise, good posture and proper ergonomics will help prevent the fatigue caused by poor body mechanics. Often it is necessary to get outside help with your structural problems. Chiropractic, massage, Rolfing (a type of bodywork involving fascia), and other types of bodywork will help you to feel better.

Chiropractic is a great way to improve your structural well-being. Frequently patients will notice that they feel much better after going to the chiropractor. Patients often report a sense of lightness and well-being that goes beyond the correction of the specific ache or pain that brought them to the chiropractor in the first place.

Most people have structural problems, slight distortions in the spine, slight muscle imbalances and tightness that are not painful. The imbalances create a kind of epicritical pain, which the patient is probably not consciously aware of. It's like a loud fan; after a while you don't notice it. When the fan is turned off, you say to yourself, "Wow, that sounds better." A chiropractic adjustment removes these slight distortions. The patient feels better, even if he or she didn't have a specific pain.

The following exercise will illustrate the importance of structural balance and how posture affects your mental attitude. Stand and breathe as if you feel depressed; slump your shoulders, hang your head down and breathe shallowly. Notice how you feel. If you do the exercise, you really begin to feel depressed. Now, stand up straight, shoulder back and head held high; breathe deeply and put a silly grin on your face. You do it and begin to feel really happy and energetic.

Neuro Linguistic Programming, or NLP, is s system of learning and communication developed by Richard Bandler and John Grinder. Many people know about NLP through Anthony Robbins, who brought it to the masses. One concept of NLP, one which is not new by any means, is the idea that we do what we do in order to *feel good*. Simply stated, anything you want in life, you want because of how it will make you feel. You want a boat or new car because it will make you feel good. If you don't feel good, NLP provides the methodology to change that. You can feel good at any time, even before you get the things you think you need. NLP is about choices, and it provides the technology to choose what emotions you want to experience. **You can feel good in an instant,** if you want to. There is an exercise for this at the end of the book. There is also a tape included in the set that will give you the tools you need to change your mood and energy level in an instant.

The exercise you just performed is an example of what Tony Robbins calls state management. It's not a new concept by any stretch of the imagination; many people do it naturally. How you carry yourself affects your mood. There is a connection between structural balance and psychological well-being. The way you carry your body affects your mood and your energy level. Chiropractors and other body workers have known this for years. To put yourself in a good mood and increase your energy, use your posture, breathing, facial expressions and body language. Simply stand straight, breathe deeply, look up and put a grin on your face. You can use your mental focus to improve the feeling. Remember a time when you felt wonderful (confident, energetic, happy—whatever emotion you wish). Mentally take yourself back to that time. Model, or recreate every gesture. Model your posture, facial expression and mental feelings. Since your brain doesn't know the difference between reality or something vividly imagined, you really do begin to feel the energy and confidence you had in the past. It's amazing; you can change your mood and energy level in an instant.

Exercise

There are benefits to exercise other than the ones that are commonly discussed by fitness experts. Increased strength, endurance and cardiovascular fitness are only the beginning. Exercise also reduces structural stress by strengthening muscles and improving posture.

Exercise improves tissue oxygenation. During exercise you breathe deeply and your heart rate increases, which increases the amount of oxygen the cells receive. Deep breathing and muscle movement during exercise also increase lymphatic circulation, improving the cells' ability to eliminate waste.

You may be so tired that a nap is a lot more appealing to you than any kind of physical activity. If you are normally sedentary, exercise will actually increase your energy. Stand up right now, and take a few deep breaths. Now, run in place for 30 seconds.

You'll notice, after doing the exercise, you have more energy than you had two paragraphs ago. Being sedentary is fatiguing. Shallow breathing and lack of muscle motion in the sedentary individual leads to poor lymphatic circulation, poor oxygenation and fatigue. Sedentary people sit there stewing in their own wastes, tired, but not ready for sleep. They may want some stimulation, but don't have the energy to do anything. What's the most likely forms of stimulus such an individual would choose? Food and TV, of course. They provide diversion, without requiring any effort.

Of course, using food and TV for diversion can make you have the dimensions of a marine mammal and be tired all of the time. You may have even created a little canyon on your end of the couch or may have an easy chair with the springs partially broken down. There is nothing quite as comfortable as a couch or chair that is contour-shaped to your rear end. The modern age is truly wonderful; you can perform less activity than a dead person and still be entertained.

A few years ago I gained 45 pounds by becoming devoted to carry-out food and bad television. My wife was pregnant, and, as a sensitive husband, I was determined to gain weight with her, pound for pound. It's easy to gain weight and feel exhausted. TV and junk food really do the job.

If you are not very active, exercise may be unthinkable. It was for me, until my landlord insisted that I lose weight or move to the first floor. He was afraid for the safety of the tenants living below me. It's a good thing we were in Chicago, because it was possible to bribe the building inspectors and keep them from condemning the building from the structural stress caused by my weight gain.

I began jogging until the department of streets and sanitation complained and threatened to have me pay for the increased repair needed to the streets and sidewalks in my neighborhood. One of the potholes I created attracted spelunkers from all over Illinois. The Illinois National Guard used it to practice rappelling. The city finally repaired the pothole after someone was injured while hang gliding across it. It made me sad to see it repaired because I had been making a nice living by selling donkey rides to the bottom.

I switched to an exercycle, which worked pretty well once we'd reinforced the seat and frame. It was surprising how much better I felt once I began exercising. I was still big enough to influence the tides when I walked near Lake Michigan, but I had a lot more energy.

The key to beginning an exercise program is to start slowly. A treadmill or exercycle is very good for pacing the intensity of your exercise. Pedal or walk slowly. Warm up this way for about 10 minutes. Gradually increase your speed until you reach your target heart rate. You will be surprised; exercise will actually energize you.

Your target heart rate is approximately 180 minus your age. This is aerobic exercise, which means that the muscles that are working are using oxygen. You do not go into oxygen debt to perform the exercise. If you go into oxygen debt, it's called, anaerobic exercise. When you exercise aerobically, you are able to converse normally while exercising. You will not be out of breath or panting. Anaerobic exercise is more of a struggle; the heart rate is higher and you do get out of breath. Moderate aerobic exercise will energize you, anaerobic exercise is much harder.

If moderate exercise at your target heart rate of 180 minus your age does not energize you, or exercise actually makes you feel worse, you may be anemic or have an underfunctioning thyroid. There are other causes, such as heart disease, but these two are the most common. Always check with your doctor before beginning an exercise program. Aerobic exercise is usually not tiring.

Anaerobic exercise is good for increasing endurance. When you start your exercise program, however, do only aerobic exercise. When you work out so hard that you are out of breath, that is anaerobic exercise. Your muscles are using more oxygen than is readily available. Anaerobic exercise can be tiring, especially if you are not used to exercising.

The first three months of your exercise program should be exclusively aerobic. After three months, add a little anaerobic exercise once or twice each week.

Whatever your exercise—rowing, cross-country skiing, biking, walking or running—take your pulse or use a heart monitor during the exercise. It is a good idea to do a variety of exercises instead of the same ones every day. Do not arbitrarily pick speed and distances.

Your pulse can be taken at your radial or your carotid arteries. The bone of the forearm that is on the same side as the thumb is called the radius. The radial pulse is found just inside (medial to) the radius, near where the wrist bends. The carotid pulse is found on either side of your windpipe. The carotid pulse is a little stronger and will be easier to find than the radial pulse. Or, if you don't mind spending a few dollars, you can buy a heart monitor.

If you still can't find your pulse, jump up and down a few times and try again. Now just count the number of beats for one minute. If you are lazy, like I am, count the beats for 15 seconds and multiply by four. If you are really out of shape, you may be surprised at how little activity it takes to get your heart rate up.

Smoking

If you smoke and you experience fatigue, thanks for buying the book, but don't you think the cause of your fatigue is obvious? Maybe not. It is not uncommon for a patient who smokes to say something like, "Do you think that if I take some ginseng I will have more energy?" It's a lot like someone who likes to hit themselves in the head with a ball peen hammer every few hours saying, "Doc, do you think that aspirin or Tylenol is better for headaches?"

When you smoke, you replace the oxygen that you should be getting with carbon monoxide and dozens of other toxic chemicals. **Smokers are prone to gastritis** and other digestive problems because the smoke stimulates enzyme production in the absence of food. Smoking also reduces the amount of oxygen that reaches the lining of the digestive tract.

Smokers are more prone to back pain than nonsmokers. Smoking destroys vitamin C, which is important for the manufacture of the connective tissue in the ligaments, tendons and intervertebral discs.

Smokers are prone to infections, especially upper respiratory infections like bronchitis. Smoking irritates the lining of the bronchi and trachea. It increases mucous production, which makes your respiratory system a breeding ground for microorganisms. Smokers are also more likely to suffer from sinusitis than nonsmokers. The list of problems that smoking causes is endless. If you smoke, you already know the problems it causes. You know firsthand from your own misery.

All smokers remember a time when they had a cold, but choked and coughed while smoking a cigarette they really didn't want, but needed. Maybe they even switched to menthol cigarettes during the course of the illness. Do you remember a time when it was 102 degrees in the shade, it felt like Rommel's Afrika Corps were having maneuvers on your tongue in dusty boots, and you still had to have a cigarette? How often do you wake up with a gut-splitting cough, producing oddly colored, hard pieces of mucous that you thought were maybe pieces of your lung? Do you wake up with your mouth feeling like you just dined on extra-absorbent kitty litter (after the cat was done with it), and still light up a cigarette? Your own misery makes the endless lecturing you receive from the people around you ring hollow, but you know they're right.

Secondhand smoke may be worth mentioning here. If you live with a smoker, or several smokers, you get all of the benefits of their habit, including sinus problems, immune suppression and, of course, fatigue.

We have some neighbors who have a daughter that is the same age as my older daughter. Recently they took her to a doctor to find out why the child was fatigued and slept so much. The doctor failed (as far as I know) to point out the obvious cause of the child's fatigue. Everyone in the house smokes, except the child, who hasn't started smoking yet.

When my daughter spends the day playing there, she gets stuffy and sleeps in the next day. The next day she is tired and congested. We always hear about cancer statistics with respect to secondhand smoke, but smoking isn't just about cancer. There are plenty of minor health problems associated with exposure to secondhand smoke. You can't expect to breathe in carbon monoxide and a dozen other noxious chemicals on a daily basis and not feel fatigued.

If you smoke, think about the people around you. This isn't about making you feel guilty. A lot of nonsmokers are pretty annoying about the subject, but that doesn't make them wrong. I used to smoke two packs of unfiltered cigarettes per day. When you smoke, you really don't notice the smoke or the smell of your living space. You tend to think nothing of it and can't figure out why nonsmokers make such a fuss about it. I know that I never did.

Do the exercise on changing habits at the end of the book to help you to quit smoking. Listen to the tape on habits. Listen to it as often as you need to, at least once each day until you successfully, completely give up cigarettes. Following the 30-day plan at the end of this part will also make it easier for you to quit smoking. Taking a multiple vitamin and some extra vitamin B complex will also make it easier for you to become smoke-free.

Alcohol

Alcohol is a toxin that damages every organ in your body. It damages the lining of the gastrointestinal tract. It can cause a condition known as leaky gut, which causes things that were never intended to get into the bloodstream to be absorbed from the digestive system. Leaky gut can cause allergies because the immune system works to defend the body against proteins and other materials that are inappropriately absorbed.

Even moderate drinking is a problem if you suffer from fatigue. Alcohol is a toxic burden on your body, and it takes energy to detoxify from drinking. During the 30-day program at the end of this section, drink absolutely no alcohol. Drinking alcohol is very fatiguing, and can undermine the benefits of the rest of the program. Even moderate drinkers are amazed at the amount of energy they have when they quit drinking. If giving up alcohol for 30 days seems like a burden to you, you may want to think about whether or not you are an alcoholic.

Nutrition is a much-neglected area in the treatment of alcoholics. Good nutrition and nutritional supplementation can be very helpful to the recovering alcoholic.

Because of problems with absorption, poor enzyme function, poor diet and destruction of cells, alcoholics are deficient in just about every nutrient there is. Alcoholics commonly suffer from depression, anxiety, tremors, fatigue and neuropathies. Many of the symptoms are directly due to the toxic effects of the alcohol; many are due to the chronic malnutrition common in all alcoholics.

Most standard nutritional texts discuss nutritional deficiencies in terms of the disease states caused by extreme deficiency. Even if a severe disease state does not exist, a slight deficiency may cause slight symptoms. For instance, if an extreme deficiency causes delirium, perhaps a slight deficiency may cause poor concentration. Here is a list of some of the nutrients that alcoholics are deficient in and the disease states caused by the deficiencies:

Vitamin A: Vitamin A is absorbed in the upper part of the small intestine. Bile salts and pancreatic enzymes are needed for the body to absorb it. Ninety percent of the body's vitamin A is stored in the liver. Zinc is needed by the body to mobilize the stored vitamin A to be used by the rest of the body.

Deficiency of vitamin A can lead to night blindness, sexual dysfunction, dryness of the eyes, skin problems and problems with the integrity of the mucosa. (Mucosa is the tissue that lines the inside of the nose, mouth and other areas inside of the body.) A lack of vitamin A and zinc can also diminish the sense of taste and smell. Hay fever sufferers who have itching eyes often find relief by taking vitamin A.

Supplementation of vitamin A can help with the growth and repair of all of the body's tissues. This is an important nutrient to the recovering alcoholic. One thing to be cautious of: An alcoholic who is still drinking, and who supplements with vitamin A will hasten the damage to his or her liver.

Toxicity can be a problem if too much vitamin A is consumed. Toxicity symptoms from overconsumption of vitamin A include constipation, emotional lability, hair loss, brittle nails, abdominal discomfort, fatigue and malaise. Beta carotene is a precursor to vitamin A and is converted to vitamin A by intestinal cells. Beta carotene is completely nontoxic. If you consume too much beta carotene, your skin may take on an orangish cast, but your normal color will return if you discontinue the vitamin. Beta carotene will not harm you.

Vitamin B complex: A study published in the British Journal of Addiction, in 1977, showed that rats deficient in vitamin B complex were more likely to choose alcohol than water. Alcoholics tend to be deficient in vitamin B complex because of poor absorption or an inadequate diet, so vitamin B deficiency may be partially responsible for alcohol cravings. It is evident that taking vitamin B complex can curb the desire for alcohol.

Thiamine (Vitamin B1): Thiamine is water soluble and nontoxic in even very large doses. The disease beriberi is caused by a thiamine deficiency. The symptoms are fatigue, anorexia, weight loss, gastrointestinal (GI) disorders and weakness. The muscles become tender and atrophied.

In the alcoholic, it is believed that Wernike's Syndrome, whose sufferers have neurological symptoms varying from mild confusion to coma is caused by a thiamine deficiency. If the thiamine deficiency persists, it leads to Korsakoff's psychosis, in which the neurologic damage is permanent.

Treatment with thiamine has been shown to improve alcoholic neuropathy. In fact, alcoholics who discontinue drinking, but were fed a thiamine-deficient diet had no improvement in their neuropathy. When thiamine was introduced to the diet, all of the subjects improved.

A study was published in the British Journal of Nutrition in 1980. Rats were given alcohol as their only fluid for one week. The rats also had varying levels of thiamine in their diet. In the following weeks they were allowed to choose between alcohol and water. Rats on a high-thiamine diet (20 mg/kg) drank only one-fifth as much alcohol as rats fed a low-thiamine diet (4 mg/kg). Rats fed a thiamine-deficient diet showed a tendency to increase alcohol drinking when intake was expressed relative to total energy intake.

Riboflavin (Vitamin B2): Riboflavin is water soluble and nontoxic. Deficiency can lead to bloodshot, itching and burning eyes that are sensitive to light. It can also lead to stomatitis and glossitis—red, smooth tongue and cracks at the corner of the mouth. Deficiency can also lead to skin lesions. Deficiency is rare in isolation, and often exists in conjunction with deficiencies in other B vitamins.

Niacin (Vitamin B3): Extreme niacin deficiency leads to pellagra, which has symptoms known as the three Ds: dermatitis, diarrhea and dementia. All parts of the digestive tract are affected. The mouth may be severely inflamed. The tongue is swollen, corroded and bright red. Diarrhea may be accompanied by vomiting. The patient may become achlorhydric (completely lacking stomach acid). Achlorhydra will cause widespread vitamin deficiencies due to lack of absorption. The achlorhydra also may lead to intestinal infection. Lack of niacin also leads to nervous system disorders including irritability, headache, insomnia, memory loss and emotional instability. In advanced stages, delirium and catatonia may develop, then convulsions, coma and death.

As with the other B vitamins, niacin deficiency doesn't usually exist alone. Also, like other B vitamins, niacin is water soluble and is non-toxic. However, large doses of niacin will produce an unpleasant flushing and itching of the skin. Prolonged and excessive doses may produce liver damage and GI irritation.

Niacin has been used to control alcohol craving. An experimental study, published in 1961, showed that alcoholics in withdrawal noted immediate abolition of almost all physical withdrawal symptoms while intravenously receiving up to 1 gram daily of diphosphopyridine nucleotide (NAD), a form of niacin, for four days. Also, an article written in the *Journal of the American Medical Association* showed that nicotinic acid (the coenzyme form of niacin reduced mortality from 90% to 14% in a large series of patients who were admitted with severe impairment of consciousness or delirium.

Pyridoxine (Vitamin B6): B6 is water soluble and nontoxic. It plays a role in protein metabolism. Deficiency may produce mental confusion, weakness, irritability and nervousness. In alcoholics, there is commonly a functional deficiency due to their inability to convert dietary B6 to the active form, pyridoxyl 5 phosphate, used by the body. This functional deficiency affects the neurotransmitters (chemicals that cause the nervous system to function). B6 deficiency can also lead to low blood sugar and poor glucose tolerance.

Folic acid: Folic acid is one of the most common deficiencies. Anemia, weight loss, apathy, anorexia, dyspnea, sore tongue, headache, palpitations, forgetfulness, paranoia, GI disturbances and diarrhea are all symptoms of folic acid deficiency. Alcohol intake reduces folic acid absorption and increases urinary excretion of folate. *The British Journal of Psychiatry* published a study that demonstrated the connection between low folate levels and depression, although researchers did not find any severity of alcohol dependence and folate levels.

Folic acid is water soluble and very nontoxic. It has been shown to prevent certain types of birth defects. The FDA sees fit to regulate the dosage of folic acid supplements available in this country. You cannot buy a dosage larger than 800 micrograms because it is possible to mask a vitamin B12 deficiency by taking large doses of folic acid.

Cobalamin (Vitamin B12): Deficiency leads to pernicious anemia, a severe megaloblastic anemia. Deficiency is usually due to a lack of production of intrinsic factor by the stomach. Intrinsic factor is necessary for the absorption of B12. Other deficiency symptoms include glossitis, degeneration of the spinal cord, loss of appetite, GI disturbances, fatigue, pallor, dizziness, disorientation, numbness, tingling, ataxia, moodiness, confusion, agitation, dimmed vision, delusions, hallucinations and eventually, psychosis.

If the deficiency is due to a lack of intrinsic factor, vitamin B12 needs to be taken by injection or by nasal gel. There is also a sublingual B12 spray that seems to be pretty effective. B12 is only found in animal products. Vegetarians who consume no B12 have an adequate supply because it is produced by intestinal microorganisms (microbial synthesis). A healthy digestive tract and normal bowel flora are necessary for vegetarians to produce vitamin B12. If they do not have normal bowel flora, they may become deficient. You don't need much B12, only a couple of micrograms per day. It's water soluble and nontoxic, even in large amounts. Alcoholics often have trouble with digestion, bowel flora and B12 absorption, and may need supplementation.

Pantothenic acid (Vitamin B5): Deficiency and toxicity are rare. It is essential for proper functioning of the GI tract. It is frequently taken as a supplement to improve adrenal function, and has improved intestinal gas in some patients. It has also been used successfully to treat paralysis of the GI tract after surgery; it seems to stimulate GI movement.

Choline: Choline is considered to be one of the B-complex vitamins. It is associated with the utilization of fats and cholesterol in the body. Choline prevents fats from accumulating in the liver. Its function is important to alcoholics, because excess alcohol consumption can cause fats to accumulate in the liver. Choline is also important for nerve function. Myelin, which surrounds many nerve fibers and is responsible for proper transmission of impulses, is a lipid (fat).

Inositol: Also considered to be a B vitamin. It helps with fat metabolism and helps reduce blood cholesterol. It is also helpful in brain cell nutrition. Large amounts are found in the brain and spinal cord.

Para-Aminobenzoic Acid (PABA): PABA stimulates the intestinal bacteria, enabling them to produce folic acid.

Vitamin C: Plays an important role in collagen formation. Connective tissue, cartilage and ligaments are made up of collagen. The symptoms of scurvy, the disease associated with vitamin C deficiency, involve connective tissue. The symptoms include anemia, joint tenderness and swelling, poor wound healing, gingivitis and tooth loss.

Vitamin C has been shown to improve the body's clearance of alcohol. It is also possible that vitamin C may prevent fatty degeneration of the liver. It is also helpful in stimulating the immune system and tissue repair. Vitamin C is an antioxidant.

Vitamin E: Is an antioxidant. It protects membranes against free radical damage, helps to prevent tumor growth, and protects the vitamin A in the body. A deficiency can affect the reproductive system, the muscular system and the nervous system.

Two-thirds of all chronic alcoholics suffer from muscle atrophy. It has been observed that alcoholics suffering from muscle atrophy also have lower serum levels of vitamin E.

While reading the symptoms of the various vitamin deficiencies, you may have noticed that they are remarkably similar to the symptoms of alcoholism. Neurological changes, muscle wasting, skin problems, ulcerations, defects in mucous membranes, depression, anxiety, confusion and craving for alcohol are all symptoms associated with alcoholism, but they can be caused by nutrient deficiency.

The symptoms of alcoholism are largely due to the fact that it leads to deficiencies in virtually every vitamin and mineral. It is obvious that these **nutrients need to be replaced in the recovering alcoholic.** Recovery is so much easier when good nutrition and vitamin supplementation are part of the regimen than it is when good nutrition is ignored.

Deficiencies in minerals are also present in the alcoholic. Magnesium deficiency has been recognized in hospitalized alcoholics. It can lead to heart, kidney and GI disorders, as well as weakness and confusion. Phosphorus deficiency can lead to symptoms similar to delirium tremens. Selenium, when taken with other antioxidants, can protect the liver from damage. Chronic alcohol consumption has been associated with zinc deficiency. Zinc is important in thousands of enzyme systems, including alcohol dehydrogenase, the enzyme which helps the body to break down alcohol. Zinc is partially responsible for detoxifying the body from alcohol. The more alcohol you drink, the less ability you have to break down the alcohol.

Amino acids are the building blocks of protein. The eight essential amino acids are those that the body cannot manufacture for itself. They must be supplied by the diet. They are often deficient in alcoholics. Amino acids are commonly precursors to neurotransmitters, which are chemicals that help the brain and nervous system to function. A precursor is the chemical that is converted into the neurotransmitter. For instance, a block of granite is a precursor to a statue.

A common outcome of deficiency in essential amino acids is depression. In fact, many psychotropic drugs mimic amino acids and other vitamin supplements. Drugs have been used more commonly than nutrients to treat depression because drug companies can own patents on drugs, but not on nutrients. In other words, there's a lot less money to be made on nutrient therapy than on drug therapy.

The FDA is trying to control the use of amino acids and other vitamin supplements. Tryptophan has already been banned, ostensibly because of adverse reactions suffered from some consumers. The symptoms were caused because of the impurity of a single brand of tryptophan imported from Japan, not because of any direct harm being caused by the tryptophan. The government's approach was a lot like banning eggs because of a single salmonella outbreak. Many people used to take tryptophan to reduce tension and to help with sleep disorders. It was an effective, drug-free way for them to take care of these problems.

A recovering alcoholic may find it discouraging to read about all the damage alcohol has done. There are two facts that are worth considering before becoming discouraged. First, people have been successfully recovering from alcoholism for years without any of this information. Second, **the human body is fairly resilient,** so if it isn't dead yet, the chances of returning to health are pretty good.

A body abused by alcohol (or any other drug), is like a 1933 Duesenberg that's been left rusting out in a field. Giving up alcohol is like putting in a new set of plugs and some fresh gasoline. It's a very well-made car, and you're amazed to find that it still runs. It may belch smoke and stall at stop signs, but it works.

Good nutrition and vitamin supplementation are like putting a little more effort into restoring the car to make a nice automobile that runs well. It's like giving the car an engine overhaul and a paint job. Alcoholism is an organic disease, and good nutrition is one of the best treatments.

People at Alcoholics Anonymous meetings have been stuffing their faces with coffee and donuts for years, completely ignoring good nutrition. In spite of this, Alcoholics Anonymous still has an impressive record for helping people maintain sobriety. Nothing here will interfere with a 12-step program. On the contrary, taking time and effort to develop healthy habits will make the whole process easier.

One of the easiest things to do is to take a good quality multiple vitamin. Not all vitamins are created equal. Thorne Research, Pure Encapsulations, Seraphin, Biotics, Nutri West and Nutricology all make a good product. These companies only sell directly to physicians, but if you have a doctor that is familiar with natural health care and nutrition, have him or her order some vitamins from one of these companies.

Multiple vitamins produced by Thorne and Pure Encapsulations are in a capsule, so there are no binders or tableting agents contained in them. Biotics' multiple vitamin is in a tablet form, but it is tableted with vegetable material and it is easily broken down by the digestive system. These supplements are easier to absorb than most vitamins you find in drug stores. The vitamins are also low dosage. For instance, a daily dosage of Thorne's multiple vitamin is six capsules. It is meant to be taken at least three times each day. A small dose, three or more times each day is absorbed by the body more effectively than taking a large dose all at once. These companies also use quality, hypoallergenic ingredients.

The companies I've mentioned are not the only ones that produce good quality vitamins. There are also companies that sell their vitamins in health food stores, which produce a decent product. Reading the label on a multiple vitamin will give you an idea of its quality. Look at the calcium and see what it is made from. It is a good indication of the overall quality of the vitamin. If you see the calcium is from dolomite, oyster shell or calcium carbonate, it is an inferior product. Minerals made from oxides and carbonates (magnesium oxide, calcium carbonate, etc.) are very low quality and poorly absorbed. Minerals that are chelated are of better quality. Gluconate is one of the cheaper chelated minerals (calcium gluconate, magnesium gluconate, etc.) If the minerals are listed as aspartate, picolinate or citrate, it is a pretty good product (example: Calcium aspartate, chromium picolinate etc.) If the manufacturers do not tell you the form of the vitamin, don't buy it.

If the product is in a capsule, it will be easier to absorb than a tablet. Also, capsules have fewer impurities than tablets. Sometimes the material used to hold the tablet together may be a source of allergens.

Vitamin B6 can be found in two forms: pyridoxine and piridoxyl-5-phosphate. The latter is the active form of the vitamin. If the B6 in your multiple is piridoxyl-5-phosphate, chances are that it is a very good quality multiple vitamin.

Vitamins are not a substitute for proper diet. Horse manure and a multiple vitamin do not a healthy body make. You need to eat properly. On the other hand, if you eat horse manure without a multiple vitamin, you are probably worse off than if you take vitamins with your horse manure. Even if you do nothing else for yourself, take a good multiple vitamin.

A recovering alcoholic should take extra vitamin B complex with the multiple vitamin; about 150 mg twice each day. If you read back over the section covering the B vitamins, you will notice that the deficiencies of the various B vitamins parallel the symptoms of alcoholism itself. Taking extra vitamin C, zinc and a multiple mineral is also helpful. If any of the deficiency symptoms are present (as listed earlier in this section), more of the vitamin that is lacking should be taken. If skin problems are present, vitamin A and zinc may be of value. If muscle tone and sexual function are problem areas, extra vitamin E may be needed. (No, taking four pounds of vitamin E each day will not turn you into the love machine. Vitamins are helpful, but they have their limits.)

Get expert advice on which vitamins are the best for you. Every individual is different, and it is difficult to create a one-size-fits-all nutritional regimen.

Sugar and the Recovering Alcoholic

Hypoglycemia is a big problem for recovering alcoholics because the body responds to alcohol much the same way that it responds to sugar. Many recovering alcoholics substitute sugar for alcohol. Alcohol is absorbed very quickly, just like sugar. It has virtually no food value, just like sugar. It's addictive, just like sugar.

Here are some of the symptoms of hypoglycemia:

- Depression
- Dizziness
- Fatigue
- Feeling weak and shaky
- Headache

Most recovering alcoholics will easily interpret these symptoms and feel the need for a drink. The symptoms of hypoglycemia are easily (albeit temporarily) relieved by a drink of alcohol.

Hypoglycemia, or low blood sugar, is also temporarily relieved by consuming sugar. Unfortunately, the consumption of sugar sets up a series of events that eventually bring back the hypoglycemia. When you eat sugar, it is rapidly absorbed, much the same way the alcohol is absorbed. The sugar is absorbed so rapidly, that the body overreacts. Insulin production far outstrips the sugar absorption, creating another hypoglycemic state within a few hours.

After giving up alcohol, many alcoholics develop a sweet tooth. They eat donuts and other sweets. Many consume soda pop at the same rate that they once consumed alcohol. There always seems to be plenty of donuts at AA meetings. Sugar can keep the recovering alcoholic on the same neurologic roller coaster as the alcohol. Although it is not as deadly as alcohol, sugar can create a number of health problems as well as make recovery more difficult. It is a safer roller coaster ride of highs and lows than is alcohol consumption, but that doesn't make it a good thing.

Ironically, sugar perpetuates the hypoglycemia that it temporarily relieves. Sugar can also cause changes in bowel pH, causing imbalances in bowel flora. This can lead to problems with nutrient absorption or leaky gut and create allergies. Sugar consumption can also cause deficiencies in vitamin B and vitamin C. It perpetuates many of the health problems caused by years of consuming alcohol.

Eating sugar may seem like a safe indulgence. In many ways it seems that sugar is an acceptable crutch that doesn't threaten your health and well-being the way that alcohol did. Many recovering alcoholics perceive that sugar consumption is making it a little easier to keep from drinking, and it is a safe substitute for alcohol.

Sugar actually makes it more difficult to stop desiring a drink. It causes blood sugar highs and lows. During the lows (that is, a hypoglycemic state), a drink can be awful appealing. The sugar roller coaster is hard on your moods, your resolve and your health. Sugar consumption can also lead to nutrient deficiency and allergies. It makes the battle to stay away from alcohol very difficult. It is a lot like denying someone sleep and trying to get them to solve difficult calculus equations.

Sugar cravings are fairly easy to control. Chewing your food thoroughly will help. Eating every two hours and snacking on fruit between meals usually will eliminate the desire for sugar. Vitamin supplementation and going on the 30-day plan will also make controlling sugar cravings much easier. Getting healthy makes recovery easier.

Sleep

Sitting here in my living room at 3:00 A.M. with my suddenly social six-month-old daughter, two things have occurred to me. First, until now, I've managed to avoid talking about one of the most obvious causes of fatigue, which is not getting enough sleep. Secondly, we were offered a lot of money for this lively infant by a band of infertile yuppies.

Obviously, **if you are going to have enough energy, you should get enough sleep.** I realize that selling your children is not always an option. You may have other reasons, such as job obligations, a too active social life, or a nocturnal neighbor who likes to play the saxophone, for not getting enough sleep. If lack of sleep is a problem for you, the best suggestion is to try to get more. You may also do the exercises for energization and stress reduction at the end of the Part 1 of the book. The tape set also has an effective sleep exercise as well as one for deep relaxation.

For many, getting to sleep and staying asleep is a problem. If it is, please come over and watch my daughter. Actually, there are some things that you can do to help yourself to sleep. For years many people took tryptophan. That was before the FDA banned it because some people became sick from a bad batch. Tryptophan is a precursor for serotonin and melotonin. Melotonin is an extract from the pineal gland. It is still available as a supplement. Many people take it and claim that it helps them to sleep.

There is some evidence that magnesium supplementation will help some people get to sleep. Calcium works for some patients. For people who have trouble falling asleep, chewing five or six calcium lactate tablets (find a brand that contains some magnesium), right before going to sleep often works.

Hypoglycemia often causes an individual to wake up and have trouble getting back to sleep. Many times eating a piece of fruit and going back to bed works.

Avoiding protein late at night helps some people to sleep. Protein contains tyrosine, an amino acid that can act as a stimulant to the nervous system. Eating a meal that is mostly carbohydrate late in the day will increase serotonin levels in the brain. Serotonin acts as a sedative. You don't want to go to bed too hungry or after having eaten too much.

If you have trouble getting to sleep, don't just lie there and worry about how much sleep you're not getting. Get up and do something relaxing. Read or work on a puzzle. When you become sleepy, go back to bed (and tell your internal dialog to shut up).

Other things you can do to improve your sleeping include avoiding stimulants such as caffeine and nicotine late in the day. If you can give them up, so much the better. Also give up alcohol. Exercise, but not too late in the day. There is evidence to suggest that **people who exercise get a better quality sleep** than those who do not. Getting up at the same time every morning makes for better sleep patterns.

At the end of the book, in the section containing the exercises, there is an exercise to help you get to sleep. The *exercise* contained in the tape set that is an excellent way to be able to *get to sleep* and *stay asleep*. Do the exercise every night. It will help you to go to sleep and to stay asleep.

The 30-Day Plan for Total Energy

Changing your habits for 30 days will eliminate your fatigue. Of course, if you want to have total energy longer than 30 days, you can stay on the program longer.

Thirty days is enough time for your new habits to become engrained and to allow your physiology to change. Also, it will be easier for you to follow a program for 30 days than it would be for you to change *forever*. Forever is a long time. If you know the program only lasts 30 days, you won't have a sense of sacrifice. People told to make permanent changes often say things like, "What?! I can NEVER have sugar again?" It's hard to stay motivated forever, but easy to stay motivated for 30 days.

Ideally, these changes will be permanent, but that's up to you. For now, just change for 30 days. People have gone on ridiculous diets for longer than that, and felt miserable, just to lose a few pounds. I personally know of people who have gone on Optifast for longer than that. Optifast is a program that allows you to only consume slop made from protein and chemicals. This 30-day program will be a joy compared to being on Optifast or on any other diet. There is no limitation to the amount of food you get to eat, just the quality. There is none of the hunger or fatigue that people get while dieting.

At the end of the 30 days you will become aware of the connection between your habits and how your feel. If you go back to your old habits and feel worse, you will understand the importance of these changes. You can then choose for yourself; either eat well or feel lousy. Most people prefer to change their habits permanently rather than feel tired.

Initially, even small indiscretions will cause your fatigue to return. As you become healthier, you will be able to indulge yourself without suffering a relapse. You may have the occasional bowl of pasta or enjoy other favorite foods at times. Birthdays, holidays and family gatherings are occasions when we all get together to destroy our health. Once your health improves you can indulge yourself on these occasions and the damage will not be too severe.

For the first 30 days, follow this program like Charleton Heston handed it to you on a stone tablet. Strictly follow it and you will be rewarded with an amazing amount of energy.

Drink at least eight, eight-ounce glasses of water each day.

Take ten deep breaths, at least three times each day: Take the breaths in the following manner: Start by forcing all of the air out of your lungs. This will make sure that you do deep diaphragmatic breathing for your next breath. After all of the air is out of your lungs, slowly inhale, filling your lungs completely. Take in as much air as you can. Pause a few seconds, then slowly exhale, taking about twice as long to empty your lungs as you did to fill them. Force all of the air out of your lungs and begin the process again.

Eat plenty of fresh fruits and vegetables: "Plenty" means that at least 70% of the volume of the food you eat should be fresh produce, and most of that should be raw. Potatoes and rice do not count as vegetables. If you have meat and a potato at a meal, you should have a large salad and a vegetable. The amount of vegetables in the meal should be about 50% greater than the amount of meat and potato. You should eat a minimum of four servings of vegetables and three pieces of fruit each day. Eat more, if you wish. If yeast is a problem for you (see the section on dysbiosis), you may need to eat more vegetables and less fruit.

Eat only whole grains: Avoid eat white, refined flour products like white bread and pasta. Eat brown rice, not white rice. Try other grains like quinoa, amaranth and millet. Oatmeal is a whole grain. Read labels on bread. Bread that looks brown and is labeled "wheat bread" usually is made with refined flour. The first ingredient listed on your bread should be whole wheat flour. Enriched flour should not be on the label. Adjectives like, Basmaji (rice) or semolina (wheat), only refer to the type of grain. They do not tell you if it is a whole grain. There are whole wheat pastas. Read the label and make sure there is no refined flour in it.

Eat slowly: Chew your food until it is liquid. Put your fork down between bites. Eating slowly improves your digestion. It is easier to digest small, thoroughly chewed particles of food than large clumps of food swallowed whole. You use a lot of energy digesting food. Taking time to chew mixes the food with the salivary enzyme amylase and makes digestion easier. If you are tired after meals and don't normally take time to chew your food, you will be amazed at how much better you feel after eating. You will also eat less. Chewing your food well also increases the absorption of nutrients.

Eat fat sensibly: Since this is not a weight-loss program, you needn't worry about how many grams of fat are in your diet. You only need to be concerned about the quality of fat that you consume.

Avoid: Deep fried food, hydrogenated and partially hydrogenated oil, roasted nuts and vegetable oils that have been extracted using heat or chemicals. Avoid cottonseed oil; cotton is not considered to be a food by the government, so the amount of pesticides used on cotton is not regulated. If you see cottonseed oil in a product, it is produced by a manufacturer who is more concerned about cost than quality.

Permitted: Good fats, have all of these that you wish. These include cold-pressed oils, extra virgin and virgin olive oil, raw nuts and avocados. Animal products can be eaten in moderation.

Absolutely avoid refined sugar: Give up candy, cake, donuts, soda pop, ice cream, cookies, sugared breakfast cereals and putting sugar on or in your food. Avoid artificial sweeteners, especially aspartame. If you must sweeten something, use a little honey or fruit juice.

Exercise aerobically for 30 minutes each day: During aerobic exercise your heart rate should be 180 minus your age. Exercise at this level is not stressful. (Of course, check with your doctor before beginning any exercise program.) During aerobic exercise you should be able to converse normally, while breathing easily. Do not exercise anaerobically during the 30 days. Do not lift weights. Do not exercise with your heart rate above 180 minus your age. Exercising anaerobically creates an oxygen debt, so you become out of breath. Anaerobic exercise is a necessary part of fitness, and can be included in your exercise program after the 30 days. Initially, during your 30-day program, it may contribute to your fatigue.

Go on a caveman diet: If the food comes in a bottle, box or a can, stay away from it. Eat foods that were available 10,000 years ago, not foods that will last 10,000 years because of all of the preservatives. Eat plenty of whole grains, fruits and vegetables. If you are not a vegetarian, eat poultry, fish and meat. If you are a vegetarian, make sure that you get enough protein by eating whole grains and legumes. Quinoa is also a complete protein.

Stay away from packaged foods, convenience foods, foods loaded with additives, canned foods, frozen foods and artificial sweeteners. Eat food in its natural state. Obviously some foods that are natural are available to us in packages, such as oatmeal and whole grain bread. The idea is to eat natural foods without additives.

Avoid alcohol and other recreational drugs.

Go on a mental diet: Give up negative thinking. Spend the next 30 days thinking only of the positive aspects of your life. People worry about their fat thighs, their crummy boss, their bitchy spouse, bills, the guy who cut them off in traffic, the fact that they didn't have a date for the high school prom or any number of other things. Even worse, they worry about things in the past, even though there's nothing that can be done about it. Worry is exhausting. Negativity causes your brain to tell you, "If things are that bad, why don't you just go take a nap?" Sleep is an escape.

It would be a good thing to spend a few minutes each morning counting your blessings. The kinds of questions you ask yourself direct your focus, so ask better questions. What is good about your life? What are you thankful for?

Most stress is a state of mind. It will sap your energy if you dwell on it.

You should be grateful that you had the price of this book (I know I am grateful that you had the price of this book); you have a warm place to read it, you are well-fed, comfortable and you are better off than most of the people in the world. You are not living in Rwanda, Bosnia or Somalia. Those people have problems that put yours to shame.

If a negative thought enters your mind, remind yourself that it can wait until next month and further remind yourself of what is good about your life. After that, look up and put a big grin on your face. That will change your focus.

Do the energization exercise every day. It's at the back of the book with the other exercises. You can also *listen* to the energization *tape*. It goes into more detail and many people *find it easier* than doing the exercises out of the book. If you don't already have them, it is strongly recommended that you get the tape set that accompanies this book.

Special Considerations

You may have some problems that need special attention. Not everything listed below will apply to all readers. Add the following to your 30-day program if they apply to you.

Keep your sinuses clear: If you suffer from sinusitis, do the following:

- Irrigate your sinuses daily.
- Purchase a HEPA filter and use it in your bedroom.
- If you have forced-air heating, get your ductwork cleaned.

If you smoke, quit: There is an exercise for habit change at the end of this section. If you have the tape set, use it. Make the effort; the reward is to begin feeling better than you've ever felt in your life. If you smoke, it is probably the single most damaging thing that you do to your health and energy. Still, many smokers may not choose not be smoke-free immediately. If you are addicted to nicotine and wish to take your time about quitting, do the 30-day program twice. First, do the other steps in the 30-day program without giving up smoking. This will improve your health and make giving up smoking easier. After 30 days, give up smoking and do the program again.

Do the habit exercise: Or use the tape. If you have special problems following any of the dietary advice, or any other aspect of the 30-day program, the "Habit Control" tape or exercise will help you.

Do the exercise to help you sleep: If getting to sleep or staying asleep is a problem for you, do the sleep exercise. Many will find that using the tape to help get to *sleep* is much *easier* than doing the exercise on their own.

Do the exercise for changing your mood: If you prefer, listen to the tape. Do this as much as is necessary, whenever you wish to improve how you feel. Practicing the exercise or listening to the tape will increase your skill in controlling your state of mind.

104

Following the program will give you *more energy* than you thought possible, and you must do everything in the program. Give up even your favorite bad habits. You may be thinking, "What? No sugar!" or, "I thought pasta was good for me." Follow the entire plan for 30 days. Do everything in the program; that includes grinning ridiculously if a negative thought crosses your mind.

People have gone on ridiculous diets and cleansing programs for longer than 30 days. It's only 30 days, you don't have to think that you'll never have junk food again. However, you'll feel so much better after 30 days that you may want to keep these good habits, especially when you find that cheating makes your fatigue return.

part two

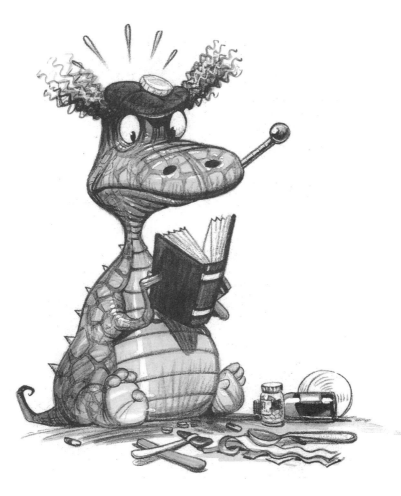

This book has been written for those who suffer from fatigue and who have not been given a satisfactory answer from their doctor about why they're tired. For some, a lifetime of bad habits may have caused a progression into poor health that needs a little more care than the 30-day plan given in Part 1. Eating sugar, for instance, will cause fatigue; but a lifetime of eating large amounts of sugar will make changes in the digestive tract that may not completely correct themselves by simply giving up sugar.

This part of the book is for those who have done the 30-day plan, or have begun the 30-day plan and their health is not perfect yet. It may take extra effort to undo the damage done by years of poor eating, being sedentary, chemical exposure and other assaults on your physiology. Changing to a healthy lifestyle is a good start. Although doing the 30-day plan will go a long way in helping you to feel better, it may be necessary to take some extra steps to ensure good health.

Back to our automobile analogy. If your car doesn't start and you've checked the gas, made sure that it was in neutral, and made sure that the battery has a charge, the car still may not start. The problem may still be relatively easy to fix. You may need spark plugs, a new Bendix spring, a new solenoid or some other relatively inexpensive repair. Similarly, problems with digestion, the endocrine system, allergies or structural balance may interfere with you enjoying excellent health and energy.

Digestion

If you were chronically ill and you could only choose one area of your body to treat, your best, first choice would be to treat the digestive system. **Problems with digestion can be the root of fatigue,** skin problems, allergies, arthritis and just about any chronic symptom that you can name.

Digesting food takes a great deal of energy. Inefficient digestion wastes energy, causes fatigue after meals and can cause malabsorption of nutrients. You could be eating a nutrient-rich diet and still not be absorbing all of the vitamins and minerals. Incomplete digestion can also cause the creation of toxic waste products that are absorbed by the body. These toxins can irritate the lining of the GI tract, and place a burden on the kidneys and liver. They can cause fatigue, much the same way that a hangover causes fatigue. A hangover is merely a toxic state.

Eating refined foods, taking drugs (prescription and otherwise), chemical additives, alcohol, environmental pollution, a diet that is deficient in fiber and nutrients, exposure to pathogenic organisms, eating too rapidly, and underproduction of hydrochloric acid and enzymes all can cause problems with digestion.

The GI tract is a muscular tube. Muscle fibers encircle it and muscle fibers run along it. The fibers pinch together to move food through the tube. That movement is called peristalsis. It's like the movement you see in a cartoon when a snake swallows an animal.

The tube runs from the mouth to the anus. Food inside the tube is still technically outside of the body. Cells lining the tube act as a barrier between the digesting food and the bloodstream. They produce enzymes to chemically break down the food. These cells also selectively absorb nutrients. The tube is in several sections. Each section is defined by the type of enzyme secreted and the type of absorption that takes place. The mouth, esophagus, stomach, small intestine, large intestine and rectum are all parts of the same tube.

Food begins its journey through the digestive tract in the mouth. Chewing is the first phase of digestion. The food is ground into small pieces and mixed with saliva, which lubricates the food. Saliva contains the enzyme, amylase, which digests carbohydrates. Chewing food thoroughly is vital to good digestion. If the food is not broken down by chewing and mixed with saliva, it will not be easy to digest.

Eating in a hurry creates problems with digestion. Let's say that you have the bologna sandwich we talked about in the food additive section, and you're in a hurry. It's a nice soft food, easy to swallow. A couple of bites and you can get it down your throat before the mustard hits your lap, letting out the occasional snort to let some air in.

The next part of the digestive tract is the esophagus. It has no enzymes, and does nothing to digest food, except to move it to the stomach. You can, however, have problems with your esophagus. Wolfing down that bologna sandwich can be the cause of some of those problems.

The esophagus has a muscular valve that separates it from the contents of the stomach. The diaphragm also helps keep the esophagus separate from the stomach. The diaphragm is the muscle that spreads across the bottom of the chest cavity and enables you to breathe. It keeps the chest and abdominal cavities separate. The esophagus travels through the chest cavity and passes through an opening in the diaphragm called the crura. It is meant to be tight around the bottom of the esophagus, keeping the stomach and esophagus separate. The separation of the esophagus from the stomach is important since the stomach contains extremely strong acid and the lining of the esophagus is not resistant to acid.

Swallowing a bowling ball-sized lump of white bread and bologna hurtles it down the esophagus toward the stomach like a boulder heading for the coyote in a Roadrunner cartoon. (Maybe it was Acme Bologna.) It hits the opening and squeezes through the crura, like Roseanne trying to get into tight lycra stretch pants.

Eating rapidly and swallowing large chunks of food can cause the crura and the muscular valve to stop being an effective barrier between the stomach and esophagus. This causes gastric reflux, or acid in the esophagus. It causes burning and discomfort. The cells lining the esophagus are not resistant to the acid in the stomach.

A hiatal hernia can also develop. This is a situation where the top part of the stomach is actually above the diaphragm, allowing stomach acid to enter the esophagus. It can cause burning and pain and can even mimic a heart attack.

Acid from the stomach is irritating to the esophagus, causing a burning sensation. The burning seems to be caused by too much acid. After all, the TV has been telling you about acid indigestion for years, so you take an antacid. The ad says, "If you eat too well, demand Di-Gel." It should say, "If you eat like an idiot, demand Di-Gel." Or, how do you spell relief? "CHEWYOURFOOD" or "USESOMESENSE."

Many people who are taking antacids actually do not produce enough stomach acid. They feel a burning sensation, not because of excess acid, but because the acid is in the wrong place. Antacids provide relief, but neutralizing stomach acid will interfere with the digestion and absorption of over 20 nutrients. This is compounded by the fact that people who inhale their food don't absorb as many nutrients as they would if they ate slowly.

If you eat a vitamin-deficient meal, and you inhale it, you don't get much nutritional value from your meal. Also eating too rapidly causes gas, bloating and fatigue after each meal. And you wonder why you're tired.

Antacids can give relief to the problem of stomach acid irritating the esophageal lining, but they do not address the cause of the problem. Eating slowly and thoroughly chewing your food often solves the problem of acid indigestion. Often acid indigestion is triggered by certain foods. Sometimes a food allergy is involved. Identify problem foods by keeping a food diary, writing down everything that you eat. Make a note each time you get an attack of acid indigestion. If a certain food is causing the attack, you will see the pattern in your diary.

There is a chiropractic technique for hiatal hernia. It really seems to work. In the past, I've had patients describe the technique to their medical doctors. They were all told that it was ridiculous and that it couldn't work. Nonetheless, many chiropractors have given hiatal hernia sufferers relief. Maybe it's the power of our dynamic personalities creating a placebo effect. Of course, if the patient experiences relief, who cares what did it?

Patients suffering with ulcers often mistake them for acid indigestion (which is one reason you should be working with a doctor and not trying to diagnose yourself from a book). Heliobacter pylori, which irritates the digestive lining, is a common cause of ulcers. There is a lab test available for Heliobacter now. If Heliobacter is present, the ulcer can usually be cured with a course of antibiotics.

The stomach, the next part of the digestive tract, is an outpouching of the tube. The stomach produces hydrochloric acid and the enzyme, pepsin, both of which work to break down protein. Of course, that huge amorphous ball of protein and starch created by swallowing a whole bologna sandwich, is very difficult for your stomach to digest. It tries, and you end up producing a lot of gas. More acid manages to get into the esophagus. Time for plop-plop, fizz-fizz.

Thoroughly chewing your food will enable the stomach to work more efficiently. If you have a piece of iron that weighs one ounce, and you place it in a beaker of acid, it will dissolve much more slowly than an ounce of iron shavings. If you thoroughly chew your food, you will eat less, absorb more nutrient and place less stress on your digestive system than if you don't.

The food leaves the stomach through the pylorus and goes into the next part of the tube, the small intestine. The small intestine is about 20 feet long and about an inch in diameter. The inner surface is ridged, giving the interior an accordion shape. The lining of the small intestine is full of fingerlike projections, known as villi, which are about a millimeter long. Each individual cell on the villi has miniature projections known as microvilli. The design of the small intestine, with the increased surface area, enhances the absorption of nutrients. Of course, swallowing a battleship-sized lump of food will make absorption less efficient.

The purpose of these projections, the villi and the microvilli, is to increase the surface area of the small intestine. If the small intestine was just a flat tube, it would have a four-square-yard area. With the added surface area of the ridges, villi and microvilli, the surface of the small intestine is more than 400 square yards, larger than a tennis court.

Alcoholism and other diseases, and even poor diet can lead to a situation known as villous atrophy, which is a flattening of the villi and the microvilli. The loss of surface area decreases the absorption of nutrients from the small intestine. This can happen from drug or alcohol use, infection or allergic reactions. In some patients, an allergy to wheat and other grains can cause irritation to the lining of the small intestine and villous atrophy. As much as half of the surface area of the small intestine can be lost, causing digestive disturbance, nutrient deficiencies and, of course, fatigue.

The first part of the small intestine is called the duodenum, which is Latin for 12. It is about 12 inches long (hence the name). This is where the pancreas adds its digestive enzymes and liver adds bile. Protease, lipase and amylase are from the pancreas. These enzymes digest protein, fat and starch respectively. Bile from the liver helps to digest fat.

The small intestine is about 20 feet long. Most of the nutrients from the meal are absorbed in the small intestine. There are three sections to the small intestine, the duodenum, which was just mentioned; the jejunum; and the ileum. The small intestine changes morphology over the course of its 20 feet. In the upper small intestine the villi are packed close together, and there is more surface area than in the lower small intestine. **Most of the absorption of nutrients occurs in the small intestine.** Carbohydrates, fats and proteins are broken down and absorbed there, as well as vitamins and minerals.

The ileocecal valve separates the large and the small intestine. It prevents the backflow of the fecal contents into the small intestines. Its function is a lot like keeping your septic tank from flowing into your well water.

Although the practice is not generally recognized by medicine, certain natural health care practitioners work on the ileocecal valve, either opening or closing it. These practitioners believe that the valve can be stuck in the open position, allowing fecal backwash into the small intestine, creating toxicity symptoms. It can also be stuck in the closed position, allowing the digested food to ferment in the small intestine, also creating toxicity. The techniques do seem to help alleviate toxicity symptoms such as headache, muscle soreness and fatigue.

The large intestine is only about five feet long, but it is much larger in diameter than the small intestine. The large intestine absorbs electrolytes and water. About half of the volume of stool consists of microorganisms. Bacteria in the large intestine produce vitamin B12 and vitamin K, which is important to blood coagulation.

Since everything you consume has to pass through the digestive tract, problems with it can cause other chronic or systemic problems. Good digestion is necessary to good health.

Hypochlorhydra

Hypochlorhydra is a state where the stomach produces less hydrochloric acid than normal. Achlorhydra is the complete absence of stomach acid. Both conditions are recognized by medicine and described in standard physiology texts; however, the medical view is that even in the absence of stomach acid, the pancreas produces enough enzymes so that digestion is nearly normal.

Most efforts by doctors to help digestion is to give substances to neutralize stomach acid. There are any number of antacids available over the counter. Doctors have commonly prescribed antacids in the past to patients suffering from ulcers; although it is now known that ulcers are caused by a bacterium and are easily cured with a course of antibiotics.

Hypochlorhydra is one of those things that is treated by doctors dealing in natural health care, but is not considered to be a problem by doctors who deal in sickness care. In this discussion, what follows is the view held by some doctors who are involved in natural health care. Just realize that not every doctor is going to agree with what is written here.

Physicians dealing in natural health care view hypochlorhydra as a problem that leads to malabsorption of minerals, poor protein digestion, vitamin B12 deficiency and even problems with bowel flora. The problems caused by hypochlorhydra can lead to a number of subclinical complaints including gas, bloating, fatigue and even depression.

Hypochlorhydra creates deficiencies in a number of nutrients. Your body needs acid in order to absorb iron, calcium and several other minerals. Vitamin B12 and essential amino acids are common deficiencies that accompany hypochlorhydra. Taking antacids can make these deficiencies worse.

People who do not produce enough stomach acid tend to dislike meat. Many vegetarians say that they feel better if they do not eat meat. A meal containing meat may cause them to have bloating, fatigue and even nausea. Chances are that these people are hypochlorhydric.

Iron deficiency anemia is a common cause of fatigue. Many times iron deficiency anemia that is not responding to iron supplementation will improve if the patient takes betaine hydrochloride (hydrochloric acid supplementation) after meals, along with their iron.

The medical model of hydrochloric acid production not being important to health and digestion is not entirely correct. There is some evidence that antacids decrease the amount of vitamin B12 that is absorbed. Also, research indicates that people who do not produce enough stomach acid have a greater tendency to be deficient in vitamin B12. This is especially common in the elderly. Vitamin B12 deficiency can cause problems with poor memory, poor concentration, fatigue and even depression. There is a possibility that some patients diagnosed with having dementia or even Alzeheimer's disease may actually be deficient in vitamin B12.

Hydrochloric acid and pepsin are necessary to break protein down into individual amino acids. Without sufficient acid, protein is not completely broken down and utilized by the body. Low stomach acid causes poor protein digestion and deficiencies in the eight essential amino acids. Amino acids are the building blocks of protein. If a protein is a freight train, the amino acids are the individual cars. Essential amino acids are those that the body can't produce for itself.

The essential amino acids are very important because they are involved with the chemistry of the brain and in the endocrine system. Deficiencies in them can cause fatigue and even depression.

Tyrosine is an essential amino acid that is necessary for the formation of both thyroid hormone and epinephrine (adrenal hormone). Both of these hormones are the body's "uppers." Without sufficient tyrosine, fatigue may be a problem.

The thyroid is the body's thermostat. The thyroid hormone controls the rate of metabolism, which is how fast you burn calories to produce energy. People suffering from hypothyroidism burn calories slowly. They are extremely fatigued, as well as having many other symptoms, including constipation, dry skin, brittle hair, frequent colds, obesity and trouble staying warm.

A person with underfunctioning adrenal glands, is similarly very tired and may crave salt, have dizziness when standing up suddenly and have other symptoms. It is possible for a lack of hydrochloric acid to affect the adrenal and thyroid glands.

Poor digestion of protein and minerals can cause people suffering from hypochlorhydra to have brittle nails and hair. It may even be responsible for hair loss. (Unfortunately, it is not the cause of male pattern baldness.)

The treatment for hypochlorhyda is to take betaine hydrochloride and pepsin after meals. Do not try to diagnose hypochlorhydra on your own. Taking hydrochloric acid supplements can cause problems in certain patients. Betaine hydrochloride can make ulcer patients feel much worse. Also, if you are taking any anti-inflammatory medication, such as aspirin, Motrin, Advil or any other nonsteroidal anti-inflammatory drug (NSAID), the supplement can cause an unpleasant burning sensation. NSAIDs irritate the lining of the GI tract. If the lining of the digestive tract is eroded or inflamed, from NSAID use or any other reason, hydrochloric acid supplements can cause irritation.

People suffering from a hiatal hernia will often experience burning and irritation when they take betaine hydrochloride. Normally the diaphragm helps separate the stomach from the esophagus. A hiatal hernia is a condition where the stomach protrudes above the diaphragm. This allows the acid that is in the stomach to irritate the lining of the esophagus. Symptoms can include chronic acid indigestion, nausea and even chest pain. Sometimes the pain is so severe that it can mimic a heart attack. Betaine hydrochloride increases the pain and burning in patients with hiatal hernia patients.

The irritation caused by betaine hydrochloride is unpleasant, but usually isn't serious. Discontinuing the supplement and taking antacids for a day or two will usually give relief.

Many of the drugs used for depression are analogs of the essential amino acids. **Frequently someone who is hypochlorhydric may be depressed as well as fatigued.** Supplementation with essential amino acids, along with hydrochloric acid supplementation sometimes helps these people.

One test to measure hydrochloric acid production is done by injecting histamine into the stomach and then taking samples of stomach acid through a tube every 10 minutes. The acid strength of each sample is then measured. This is an extreme measure.

There is also a machine that will test stomach acid levels, called a Heidleberg gastric analyzer. The test is easier on the patient and is usually performed right in the doctor's office. The patient swallows a capsule, which is a tiny radio transmitter. The transmitter measures the pH as it travels through the GI tract and sends the information to a receiver outside of the patient (easier for the technician to read that way).

Hypochlorhydra is fairly common. Some physicians treat it without using either of the above tests. If the patient doesn't have an ulcer or hiatal hernia, or is not taking antiinflammatory medication betaine hydrochloride rarely causes any trouble.

Hypochlorhydra can be at the root of other digestive problems. It can cause leaky gut, malabsorption and even dysbiosis.

Dysbiosis

Residing in the large intestine are large numbers of microorganisms. Half of the volume of your stool consists of microorganisms. Some belong there and some do not. Dysbiosis refers to the absence of normal bacteria, overgrowth of pathogenic organisms or bacteria growing in an area of the digestive tract that normally has no bacteria.

Most people are familiar with dysbiosis from Dr. William Crook's book The Yeast Connection. Crook's idea is that people suffering from many chronic health problems, including allergies, headaches, fatigue, body aches, asthma and skin problems, and patients who are just plain sick, have a problem with proliferation of yeast in their large intestine.

Dysbiosis can also refer to parasites growing in the large intestine. Parasites can cause problems very similar to those that yeast causes. Because yeast is so much more common than parasites, often people go through regimens to get rid of yeast, when, in reality, their problems are caused by amoebas or other types of parasites.

Microorganisms growing where they do not belong is also a form of dysbiosis. In a sense, the word dysbiosis can refer to ulcers caused by Heliobacter pylori. There is a theory the Crohn's disease is caused by overgrowth of normal bacteria in the small intestine. This is dysbiosis, since bacteria do not belong in the small intestine.

Yeast

Candidiasis is not an aversion to the music of Tony Orlando. Otherwise it would be declared a national epidemic and the price of garlic would go through the roof. Candidiasis is another word for yeast infestation in the bowel. Yeast exist, to some extent, in everyone's digestive tract. The normal bowel flora, bacteria that belong in the bowel, keep the yeast in check. If the normal bacteria die, yeast can proliferate, causing candidiasis. It can lead to allergies, leaky gut and digestive disturbances. Generally candidiasis undermines health. Patients are not only fatigued, but they may also have other symptoms such as headaches, hypoglycemia, sinus problems, irritable bowel, nausea and other digestive problems, joint pain, rashes, hives and other skin problems. Smoke and fumes often bother them. They often suffer from the just-plain-sick syndrome; feeling miserable, but unable to get a definite diagnosis from traditional physicians.

Candida patients tend to feel worse in damp and dark places. This is because mold grows in moist dark places, and candida patients tend to be sensitive to mold. Also, smoke and perfume can cause a flare up of symptoms. Many people who now have a problem with yeast and mold often have a history of eating a lot of refined food or frequent treatment with antibiotics. Eating a highly refined diet, with lots of sugar and refined white flour nourishes the yeast and kills the normal bacteria. Frequent use of antibiotics can lead to yeast proliferation in the large intestine.

Antibiotics kill normal bowel bacteria, but leave the yeast unmolested. Repeated ear infections as a child, antibiotic therapy for acne as a teenager, recurrent bladder or sinus infections or bouts of strep throat are common reasons for antibiotic therapy. Many people who do not now enjoy good health had a period in their life when they took a lot of antibiotics.

The large intestine has wildlife in it, much like a forest or any other ecosystem. If the wolves are killed off, the forest becomes overgrown with deer and rabbits. In the intestine, if the normal bacteria are killed off, the intestine becomes overgrown with yeast and pathogenic bacteria.

Also, repeated bouts of antibiotic therapy tend to create *super bugs*, or bacteria that are antibiotic resistant. Antibiotics, while curing the immediate problem, predispose patients to future infections by disturbing the normal floral balance and by creating antibiotic-resistant strains of bacteria. This is on top of the fact that frequent use of antibiotics can cause yeast overgrowth in the large intestine.

Yeasts are one-celled organisms. They are like little chemical factories. They feed on carbohydrates, especially sugars. They release waste material, which contributes to the taste of foods like cheddar cheese, vinegar and beer. In the intestines, the waste products of the yeast can create problems. They irritate the intestinal lining and they kill normal bacteria, causing leaky gut and making the dysbiosis worse. The chemical toxins from the yeast are also absorbed by the body and can cause intolerance for smoke, perfumes and other chemicals by overloading the body's mechanism to remove them.

Yeast and their chemical waste products eventually challenge the integrity of the intestinal wall leading to a condition known as leaky gut. This can cause allergies. In leaky gut, the intestine is not an effective barrier. Material in the intestines are technically outside of the body, with the intestinal wall acting as a barrier between it and the bloodstream. In leaky gut, the intestinal wall's effectiveness as a barrier is compromised and things that belong outside of the body are absorbed into the bloodstream.

Much of the therapy for candidiasis concentrates on killing the yeast. If you read Dr. Crook's book, *The Yeast Connection*, you will notice that almost all of his patients take Nystatin to kill the yeast; *and* they are on a very strict diet.

Sometimes yeast proliferation can be brought under control without as heavy-handed an approach as some of the antiyeast programs. Taking Nystatin long term is not usually necessary. In fact, many patients effectively handle their yeast problem without the use of drugs.

One problem with taking Nystatin long term is that not all strains of candida are sensitive to it. Also, yeast can mutate and develop tolerance to antifungal substances. Anything that you take to kill yeast will eventually lose its effectiveness. Another reason that Nystatin is not always effective is the fact that yeast can exist in several forms, some of which are more virulent than others. In its more virulent state, yeast can invade the wall of the intestine, making it harder to treat. Nystatin, which does not get into the bloodstream, may not be effective. Nyzoral, a drug that does enter the bloodstream is sometimes used to kill the more virulent form of yeast. There are herbs and other natural substances that will kill the more tenacious form of yeast. These include caprillic acid, undecenoic acid, grapefruit seed extract and garlic.

An effective strategy for bringing candidiasis under control is to take one of these substances for about a month and then switch to another one. Garlic and undecenoic acid are also absorbed into the bloodstream and can kill the more virulent forms of yeast.

There is a product made from oregano, called ADP. It is manufactured by a company known as Biotics. Clinically, this substance seems to be a very effective antifungal. It also seems to kill much more than just yeast. It can kill pathogenic bacteria, possibly some parasites and, unfortunately, normal bacteria.

If you take ADP, as with any antiyeast regimen, replacing the normal bacteria is very important. Take acidophilus and bifidus bacteria for at least 60 days after you finish taking ADP. Also take fructo-oligo saccharides and short chain fatty acids. These substances nourish normal bacteria, without feeding yeast or pathogenic bacteria. Strictly avoid refined carbohydrates like sugar and white flour. Sugar and starch feed yeast and suppress the growth of normal bacteria.

There are many people who are given a diagnosis of candidiasis who are avoiding yeast. This isn't necessary unless they are also allergic to yeast. Yeast overgrowth in the intestine and yeast allergy are not the same thing; however, they can exist together.

In treating candidiasis, it is more important to treat the body that has the yeast, rather than just treating the yeast. Frequently patients undergoing treatment for candida will still experience symptoms and think that the yeast is still there. In reality, the symptoms are from nutrient deficiencies, leaky gut or allergies. Dealing with all of the health issues is a much more effective way of treating candidiasis patients than becoming obsessed with killing the yeast.

In a healthy bowel, the normal bacteria keep the yeast in check. Taking lactobacillus and bifidus bacteria is helpful, but often these organisms don't survive in a yeast-infested gut. Changing the environment of the bowel will promote the growth of normal bacteria and keep the yeast in check.

Something as simple as eating vegetables will help balance the bowel flora, eliminating yeast and nurturing the normal bacteria, which feed on vegetable fiber. Make a raw, chopped salad two or three times each day. Take any raw vegetables that you like and chop them in a food processor. You can season them with salt, pepper, oil and lemon. It is tasty and good for your digestion.

Strictly avoiding refined sugar and white flour is vital. If yeast is a problem, you will not return to health if you persist in eating refined foods. Yeast feed on carbohydrate and really thrive on refined carbohydrate.

Vitamin supplementation is also important, since many of the symptoms suffered by candida patients are the result of nutrient deficiency. Everyone is unique. There is no single candida nutrient program. A good multiple vitamin, some vitamin B complex and vitamin C are a good start. Biotin, a B vitamin suppresses yeast growth and helps normal bacteria to grow. Trace minerals are especially important. Sensitivity to smoke and perfume is one of the more common symptoms of candida patients. Taking a trace mineral, molybdenum, often alleviates this symptom.

Testing stool samples for yeast is a good way to monitor the efficacy of your treatment. Great Smokies Labs in Ashville, North Carolina and Meridian Labs in Oregon both will test stool samples for yeast. Testing can also keep you from persisting in taking herbs or even drugs unnecessarily.

Candidiasis is a controversial subject. Many physicians don't believe that it even exists. A recent study in a respected medical journal had subjects suspected of suffering from candidasis taking Nystatin. No other type of therapy, nutritional supplementation or diet was included in the study. The study concluded that Nystatin was of no value to these patients. Of course the doctors who ran this study are now gearing up to study the phenomena of frogs who are hard of hearing and unable to jump.

Effectively treating candidiasis involves a multifaceted approach. Modern medicine with its propensity toward single-element treatments, tends to disbelieve the idea that Candida albicans can cause systemic disease. Of course at one time, respected physicians thought that Pasteur's ideas were a lot of nonsense.

Parasites

Parasitic infection can lead to the following symptoms: chronic fatigue, abdominal pain and cramps, anorexia, autoimmune disease, distention, fever, food allergy, gastritis, inflammatory bowel disease, leaky gut, irregular bowel movements, irritable bowel disease, low back pain, itching anus, rashes, hives, weight loss, arthritis, bloody stools, colitis, Crohn's disease, diarrhea, dysentery, flatulence, foul-smelling stools, headaches, malabsorption, vomiting and even depression. Many times patients who are suspected of having cadidiasis actually have parasites.

One of the most common misconceptions about parasites is the idea that they are extremely rare. They are much more common than most people realize. Many physicians think of parasitic infection as a disease of the tropics or of the third world. Although parasites are more common in the tropics, they also exist in the United States. We have truly become a world village. People from the tropics, and from the rest of the planet, live in the United States. We import produce from all around the world. People can travel halfway around the world in a single day. People from the United States regularly go to the tropics. This blending of populations includes blending of microbial populations. We are no longer protected from parasitic infection by winter and distance.

Estimates vary, but between **15% and 30% of Americans have a parasitic infection.** Great Smokies Diagnostic Laboratory reports that 30% of the samples it tests contain parasites. This number may be higher than the general population since people tend to send samples to Great Smokies when they have gastrointestinal complaints.

Parasites that infect the human intestinal tract are either protozoa (one-celled organisms) or helminths (worms). They are found by testing stool samples. Even laboratories that specialize in testing stool samples, like Meridian Labs and Great Smokies, can miss finding a parasite, although they do a better job than most hospitals. Frequently, several types of samples are used. Samples of regular bowel movements, bowel movements taken after using a laxative (purged stool sample) and by swabbing the area around the anus (to find eggs left by worms). Finding parasites is very difficult. The technician literally has to sort through poop to find something microscopic in size. (I don't know what Great Smokies pays, but these guys can't be making enough money.)

Most hospital labs do not take parasites very seriously. You may be asked if you've been to the tropics. You may tell them no, but you've been to Jamaica Joe's Cajun Sushi Bar on the West Side of Chicago and that you've had gas and diarrhea for the last eight months. Your vinyl upholstery is starting to crack and blister, and no one will sit in a car with you. In fact, on the way to the doctor, the cab driver paid you to get out. The lab may reluctantly agree to take your sample, since they've just gotten a patient from Jamaica Joe's who's been on IV fluids for the last three weeks. They test your stool, without a purged sample or a peri-anal swab, and it comes out negative. You are given some Kaopectate, a clothes pin for your spouse's nose and the doctor's condolences.

Just because a laboratory didn't find a parasite doesn't mean that one doesn't exist. There is a certain amount of skill required in preparing and reading the sample. Taking different types of stool samples is also very important. Sometimes several stool samples test negative before a parasite is actually found. It is best to use a laboratory that specializes in finding parasites and that takes parasitic infection seriously.

While it is true that the most common symptoms of parasitic infection are abdominal pain, gas and diarrhea, it is possible to have a parasitic infection without these symptoms. A person infected with parasites may simply be fatigued or depressed. Sometimes the parasite only causes gastrointestinal problems at one stage of its life cycle, so that the patient only experiences gas, abdominal pain or diarrhea occasionally.

Bowel Ecology

Good bowel ecology is necessary if you are to have enough energy. Poor bowel ecology can lead not only to fatigue, but to many other health problems as well. Even diseases like rheumatoid arthritis, ankylosing spondylitis and other autoimmune diseases seem to be caused by bowel problems. Individuals with these diseases form antibodies to bacteria in the intestine. These antibodies attack the individual's own tissue, creating the autoimmune disease.

Normal flora in the large intestine are necessary to keep yeast and pathogenic bacteria in check. Normal flora compete with yeast and pathogens for nutrients, and they produce natural antibiotics. Normal flora also break down toxins produced by the yeast and pathogens.

The environment of the colon determines what kind of microorganisms will live there. The pH of the bowel is very important. The stool is supposed to be slightly acidic. A high (alkaline) pH suppresses the normal flora. Hypochlorhydra is one cause of an alkaline pH in the bowel. Diets that are low in fiber and high in sugar and fat can also create a high bowel pH. Yeast and pathogenic bacteria will thrive in a high pH, at the expense of normal bacteria. Drugs, especially antibiotics, steroids and alcohol can contribute to yeast overgrowth.

Poor bowel ecology, or dysbiosis, causes an increase in toxic chemicals in the bowel, such as ammonia, phenols, amines, nitrites and aldehydes. The toxic chemicals of the pathogens further suppress the growth of normal bacteria and irritate the lining of the intestine. Pathogenic bacteria can even increase estrogen levels and thereby play a role in PMS and breast cancer.

The loss of normal bacteria also causes a loss of nutrients that they produce, including vitamin B12, vitamin K and other substances such as short chain fatty acids. These are meant to nourish the lining of the large intestine. The result can be fatigue, anemia, neurological problems, easy bruising and leaky gut.

In an alkaline bowel more ammonia is absorbed than in a bowel with normal pH. Ammonia inhibits oxidative metabolism in the brain. Absorption of ammonia and other toxic chemicals can lead to a deep fatigue that many patients describe as being like a hangover. These patients are so fatigued, that no amount of sleep seems to make them feel better. They have a foggy feeling and poor concentration. Clinical ecologists call this feeling *brain fag*. (Although many believe that brain fag is a term used to describe Mensa members who live on the North Side of Chicago and like show tunes, it is actually short for fatigue.)

Brain fag is a common complaint of patients with food allergies, dysbiosis and chemical sensitivity. It is primarily caused by toxicity. Toxins from yeast, pathogenic bacteria, parasites, toxins absorbed from leaky gut and chemical debris from an overworked immune system can all cause brain fag. If you've ever had a bad hangover, you have a good idea of what brain fag feels like.

Dysbiosis can also refer to normal bacteria living in the small intestine, where they don't belong. There is some speculation that Crohn's disease is caused by overgrowth of normal bacteria in the small intestine.

Crohn's disease, or regional ileitis, is an inflammatory disease of the small intestine. Sections of the small intestine become irritated. As the inflammation persists, the intestine narrows and becomes hard. These patients often suffer from severe abdominal cramping and other bowel disturbances. Sometimes the bowel becomes so narrow and loses so much of its elasticity that sections of it must be removed surgically.

Crohn's disease is very complicated. In some cases, Mycobacterium have been involved. These patients also have increased intestinal permeability (leaky gut—see the next section). Their white blood cells often overreact to Candida albicans and to normal flora. They are often deficient in zinc, selenium and magnesium. Supplementation with these minerals is often beneficial.

Crohn's patients often benefit from a diet that is low in sugars. Also, eating meals that consist of a single food is beneficial. Finding and avoiding food allergens helps to alleviate the symptoms of Crohn's disease. Gluten is a common allergen that Crohn's suffers react to.

Many Crohn's patients benefit from a diet known as the Specific Carbohydrate Diet, presented in Elaine Gottschall's book *Food and the Gut Reaction*. The diet limits the type of carbohydrates patients can eat. It's goal is to limit microbial growth in the intestine. No grains, potatoes, soy beans or chick peas are permitted. If you suffer from Crohn's disease or ulcerative colitis, this book is worth getting. The diet doesn't cure everyone, but those it does help often have a *permanent* remission of symptoms, without having to stay on the diet forever.

Ulcerative colitis is similar to Crohn's disease. Crohn's is a disease of the small intestine, while ulcerative colitis is a disease of the large intestine. These patients often have amoebic infection (parasites). Frequently, they will have had amoebic dysentery in the past. A pathogenic bacteria known as Clostridium dificile is often involved. Testing the stool for parasites or pathogenic bacteria is advisable. Patients often do well by giving up dairy products. High doses of fish oil sometimes help to control the inflammation of ulcerative colitis. Eighteen capsules per day of Max-EPA (fish oil) have been given in clinical trials with encouraging results.

Another clinical trial involved treating ulcerative colitis patients by killing all of the bowel flora with massive doses of antibiotics. The patients were then given a mixture of normal bowel flora. Eighty-six percent of these patients went into remission. This is not a practical treatment, but it does show a definite connection between dysbiosis and ulcerative colitis.

There may be a variety of causes for diseases like Crohn's and ulcerative colitis. The specific carbohydrate diet will help many of these patients, but not all. Finding allergies, balancing bowel flora, killing pathogens and nutrient supplementation are all possible treatments.

Crohn's disease and ulcerative colitis are just two examples of diseases that may be caused by dysbiosis. There is evidence to show that psoriatic arthritis, ankylosing spondylitis, psoriasis, eczema and rheumatoid arthritis are also linked to dysbiosis.

Problems with the gut flora can go beyond fatigue. Skin trouble, arthritis, digestive problems, autoimmune diseases, PMS and even cancer can be linked to dysbiosis.

Leaky Gut

Material in the digestive tract is still technically outside of the body. The cells lining the GI system break the material down and selectively absorb nutrients. These cells act as a barrier between the bloodstream and the digestive material. Alcohol, drugs, a highly refined diet, environmental poisons and toxins resulting from dysbiosis, all irritate the cells lining the intestinal tract. Over time the cells become ineffective as a barrier against toxic molecules, undigested protein and even microorganisms. If the situation continues unchecked, large molecules, which would normally remain in the intestine, enter the bloodstream. Once there, these large molecules are not recognized as food, but as foreign invaders, triggering a response from the immune system. This is known as *leaky gut*.

Protein is important to the immune system. Proteins are large molecules, much like a freight train. The train is made up of smaller molecules, analogous to the cars of the train. These smaller molecules are called amino acids. There are 22 of them. Eight of the 22 are essential; they have to be provided externally because the body can't manufacture them. In a healthy digestive system, any protein eaten is absorbed as individual amino acids. If it is not completely broken down, a healthy intestine will keep it out of the bloodstream. In leaky gut, incompletely digested protein, called peptides, are absorbed.

Peptides are groups of amino acids linked together. They are large enough to be noticed by the immune system, which works by recognizing protein that doesn't belong in the body. Protein provides the structure of the cell; that is, its framework. It is very much like the 2 x 4 studs that make up the frame of a house.

The structure of invading organisms, like viruses and bacteria, have their own protein frame. Your immune system recognizes the difference between the framework of your own cells and the framework of the invaders' cells.

When an invader is recognized, the cells of the immune system attack it. They release chemicals, like histamines and kinins, to destroy the invaders. White blood cells, known as phagocytes absorb the invaders. There is chemical warfare, producing free radicals. Symptoms experienced when the body is sick, such as fever, runny nose, muscle aches and other symptoms, are usually due to the actions of the immune system.

128

When a peptide is absorbed by someone suffering from leaky gut, the immune system doesn't know the difference between it and an invading virus. Chemical warfare begins. The nose runs, sinuses fill up and the sufferer becomes fatigued. An allergy develops. If long-term exposure occurs, the individual may suffer from asthma, migraines, severe fatigue, colitis, immune suppression, frequent infections, eczema and other skin problems or just about any chronic health problem you can name.

People who suffer with these symptoms have many allergies. Some of the allergies they are aware of, others, they are not. Also, those who suffer from the just-plain-sick syndrome usually have some kind of digestive problem. A combination of leaky gut and hypochlorhydra is very common. Hypochlorhydra causes incomplete protein digestion, thus forming many peptides. It can also cause an imbalance in the bacterial flora, leading to leaky gut. Leaky gut causes the peptides to be absorbed, putting the immune system in disarray.

Leaky gut may partially explain the connection between autoimmune diseases and problems with the digestive tract. Autoimmune diseases often result from immune system responses that have gotten out of control and begun to attack the body's own cells. For instance, some evidence exists that some cases of rheumatoid arthritis are the result of the body being hypersensitive to a pathogen in the bowel. The immune system attacks the bacteria, but the bacteria has similarities to their own cartilage. The immune system then attacks the joint cartilage, resulting in red, swollen, painful and distorted joints.

There is a laboratory test available for leaky gut. It is called the intestinal permeability test and is available through Great Smokies Diagnostic Laboratory. The test involves drinking a solution of two sugars, lactulose and mannitol. Mannitol is a small molecule and is usually easily absorbed. Lactulose is a large molecule and is not broken down or absorbed.

After the patient drinks the solution, the urine is tested for the presence of the two sugars. Mannitol should be absorbed by everyone. If it is not present, or if it is present in low levels, malabsorption is a problem. Lactulose should not be absorbed by a healthy intestine. If it is present in the urine after drinking the solution, the patient has leaky gut.

What to Do If Digestion Is a Problem

It is hard to tell what exactly is wrong with your digestion simply by your symptoms. Gas, bloating and abdominal pain can be the result of hypochlorhydra, yeast, parasites, enzyme deficiency or simply eating too rapidly. Fatigue can be the result of allergies, nutrient deficiency, leaky gut, yeast or parasites. Loose stools can be caused by yeast, parasites, pathogenic bacteria or enzyme deficiencies. Parasitic infection, poor digestion and poor absorption can be present even without obvious symptoms.

There is an overlapping of these problems and they often exist together. Someone who is hypochlorhydric, for instance, has a better chance of having dysbiosis than someone with normal stomach acid production. One of the roles of stomach acid is to prevent dysbiosis. Few microbes can survive the pH of a normally functioning stomach. If you have parasites, it is possible that you do not produce enough stomach acid.

Low stomach acid also causes the general pH of the bowel to be alkaline, creating an environment that favors yeast over normal bacteria. Also, people with low stomach acid tend to overeat and to crave sugar. Alkaline bowel and sugar consumption is a recipe for candidiasis.

Toxicity and poor nutrient absorption can cause underproduction of hydrochloric acid and other enzymes. It is a cycle. Low hydrochloric acid can lead to dysbiosis; dysbiosis can lead to leaky gut and poor nutrient absorption; poor nutrient absorption can lead to low production of hydrochloric acid. Dysbiosis can cause the immune system to overwork and lead to food allergies, which makes digestion even worse. Hypochlorhydra, dysbiosis, food allergies, leaky gut and poor nutrient absorption often exist together.

If you suffer from gas; bloating; fatigue after meals; loss of desire for meat; sugar or bread cravings that are hard to control; or food allergies, the problem probably has its roots in your digestive system. You may find it discouraging because after reading this, you can't be sure of what exactly is wrong with your digestive system. Is it hypochlorhydra? Is it dysbiosis? Is it leaky gut? Is it a parasite, or yeast? How do you tell the difference?

Dr. George Goodheart, the man who is credited with the initial development of applied kinesiology, has a good analogy that applies to how people commonly view health. He says that if you have a zebra in your kitchen that is tearing up the place, breaking things and having a bowel movement on your kitchen floor every hour, some people are very reassured to know that the zebra's name is Fred.

If you have symptoms but don't know the name of the disease, it is very disturbing. Once a doctor gives a name to the disease, you are somehow reassured, even if not much can be done for it. The doctor can tell you that you have irritable bowel, colitis or gastritis, and that satisfies most people. Sometimes drugs are given to manipulate the symptoms, but a cause and a solution are never found. Wouldn't it be great to find out why "Fred" is there? And isn't it more important to get rid of him than it is to know his name?

There are some basic changes you can make in your diet and lifestyle that will improve poor digestion. Some of these are repeated from the 30-day plan in the first part of this book. In fact, you may have tried the 30-day plan and found that your digestion has improved somewhat. However, if the 30-day plan hasn't made your digestion quite perfect yet, you may try the following:

Chew your food until it is liquid: This is the single most important thing you can do to improve digestion. It is easier to digest tiny particles of food than it is to digest big pieces of poorly chewed food. Also, enzymes in the saliva begin the digestive process.

Make and drink fresh vegetable juices: Vegetables are high in vitamins, minerals enzymes and antioxidants. Vegetable juice gives you a nutrient-rich diet without having to take a lot of vitamin pills or eat a lot of food. Chlorophyll from green vegetables helps heal the bowel lining and repair leaky gut. Drinking fresh vegetable juices is a great way to get vitamins in their natural state. I use a Vita mix, which is sort of a blender with a supercharger on it. I swear you could put gravel in a Vita mix, throw in a little water, and turn it into juice (stone juice, sounds like something you'd have on the caveman diet). You can put cabbage, spinach, carrots or any other vegetable into the Vita mix and liquefy it. Juice made in the Vita mix has the added advantage of still containing all of the fiber.

Eat vegetables: Eat at least five or six servings of vegetables each day. Also, have a chopped salad at least two times each day. Cabbage is a good base because it helps to heal leaky gut. Add any other vegetables that you like. The fiber from the vegetables will nourish the normal bacteria in your bowel. The fiber in vegetables stimulates the production of mucous in the intestine, which inhibits the attachment of trophozytes (form of parasites). Normal bacteria will produce nutrients that will help nourish and heal the bowel lining. Normal bacteria also produce natural antimicrobial substances that suppress the growth of yeast and pathogenic bacteria. It is best to eat raw vegetables, but if they give you gas, eat them steamed or boiled.

132

Take two garlic capsules after each meal: Garlic kills yeast, pathogenic bacteria and inhibits the growth of many parasites. It does not harm the normal bowel flora. Garlic is also an excellent antioxidant. There are various herbs and drugs that are better for killing yeast and parasites, but they should be taken under a physician's care after a specific diagnosis has been made. Garlic will not harm you (unless you are allergic to it), and it is beneficial to your health in many other ways.

Take normal bowel flora: This can be purchased in a health food store. Get a refrigerated powder with acidophilus and bifidus bacteria. Take 1/4 teaspoon of the powder mixed in water, three times each day, after meals. You can even mix it into your vegetable juice.

Absolutely avoid refined sugar and white flour: Sugar and white flour change the bowel pH and feed yeast in the intestine. Avoid anything that is refined; eat only whole grains.

Go on a caveman diet: Yep, going to the drive-in frequented by Fred Flintstone and eating a slab of ribs big enough to tip your car over is a sure cure for digestive problems. You know this really means that you should avoid additives and eat foods the way nature provides them.

This advice can be followed without causing any harm. It will be of benefit to anyone, even if they do not have problems with digestion. People following this advice often experience dramatic improvements in their digestion. If your problem is too severe, get professional help.

Sometimes yeast infestation is so severe that it is necessary to follow a more aggressive regimen. Many times it is necessary to specifically diagnose what is wrong. Often an antiyeast program will be unsuccessful because the problem is caused by a parasite. A physician who understands about yeast, dysbiosis and leaky gut has many tools at his or her disposal to diagnose and treat you. With the information attained from lab tests, the physician can then pursue a more aggressive treatment. If parasites are found, frequently both drugs and herbs are used to bring them under control. It is often very difficult to get rid of parasites.

A typical antiparasitic product contains grapefruit seed extract, artemesia (wormwood), gentian and berberine. Undecenoic acid and caprillic acid are often used to fight candidiasis. These substances are available in health food stores. If, however, you've done all of the dietary suggestions in this section and are still having trouble, don't experiment with herbs and vitamins. Get some help and have your problem properly diagnosed and treated.

Some of the issues you can explore with your physician are as follows:

Leaky gut: Quercitin is a bioflavenoid that will help heal leaky gut. Another commonly used substance is spirulina, which is also known as blue-green algae. Spirulina contains quercitin. It also has a lot of other nutrients, including chlorophyll. Licorice also helps to heal leaky gut; it can be taken in capsules or as licorice tea. Be careful taking licorice, it can raise your blood pressure. It is also a stimulant to the adrenal gland and it may not be a good idea to take it if functional hypoadrenia is a problem. Cabbage juice helps heal leaky gut, as do chlorophyll capsules.

Candidiasis: People who have had many courses antibiotic therapy for acne, repeated ear or bladder infections, or strep throat often suffer from candidiasis. Although they may suffer from many chronic complaints, the most telling symptoms are sensitivities to smoke and perfume and a worsening of symptoms in damp, moldy places. Garlic is useful against Candida albicans, but it is a good idea to change the antifungal substance every four to six weeks. Other useful antifungals are: grapefruit seed extract, berberine, undecenoic acid, caprillic acid and ADP. Killing the yeast often causes an initial worsening of symptoms. This usually improves after a few days. Limiting the consumption of carbohydrates is also helpful. There are more aggressive treatments available, but they should be followed under a physician's care.

Normal bowel flora: Not having enough normal bacteria is also a form of dysbiosis. Taking acidophilus and bifidus bacteria will only be effective if the environment of the bowel is favorable to their growth. There are two supplements that encourage normal bowel flora to grow—fructo-oligo saccharides and short chain fatty acids. These substances feed the normal bacteria but not the yeast and pathogens.

Parasites: You should not try to get rid of parasites without a diagnosis and advice from a physician. Sometimes a combination of drugs and herbs are needed to get rid of these tenacious microorganisms. Antiparasitic drugs are pretty heavy duty and often have side effects. Many herbs and natural substances are effective. Berberine (the active ingredient of goldenseal), gentian, artemisia (wormwood), citrus seed extract and even garlic are have been effective against parasites. Stay out of Jamaica Joe's Cajun Sushi Bar.

Carbohydrates: Carbohydrates, especially refined carbohydrates, are often a problem for people suffering from candidiasis and other forms of dysbiosis. Elaine Gottschall's Specific Carbohydrate Diet is primarily designed to fight dysbiosis.

Carbohydrate intolerance, or hyperinsulinism, may be worth mentioning here. Phil Maffetone writes about carbohydrate intolerance in his book *In Fitness and in Health*, which, by the way, is a great book. Read it if you work out, are involved in sports or are interested in exercise at all. In the book, Maffetone doesn't speak of carbohydrate intolerance with respect to yeast or dysbiosis, but rather as a function of the patient's ability to utilize carbohydrates. Patients who are carbohydrate intolerant may suffer from fatigue, poor concentration, low blood sugar, intestinal bloating, increased fat storage (especially pot belly or large buttocks), increased blood pressure and depression.

Maffetone's book contains excellent information about sports performance and nutrition. It is not about dysbiosis; however, his approach to patients with carbohydrate intolerance may be valuable to patients with candidiasis.

Find a doctor to monitor your progress with this test. For two weeks do not eat any carbohydrate, except for a piece of 100% whole grain bread at breakfast. Eat no products that contain grain such as bread, rolls, rice oatmeal, pasta, pancakes, cereal and muffins. Eat no sweets, including products that contain sugar like ketchup and other condiments. Avoid fruit and fruit juice. Eat no potatoes, corn or beans. Also avoid milk and yogurt.

You can eat meat (except for cold cuts), poultry, fish, eggs, cheese and any vegetables (except for corn, potatoes and beans). You should also eat as much food as you want. This is only for two weeks, but you must go the full two weeks without breaking discipline.

If, after two weeks on the program, you've lost weight, improved your mood, began bloating less or have other significant improvements in your health and well-being, you probably need to be eating fewer carbohydrates. After the two-week test, gradually add carbohydrates to you diet. Don't add any sugar or refined carbohydrates. Add a potato or a serving of beans. See how you feel for the next couple of days. If your symptoms do not return, you can increase your carbohydrate intake a little more.

If your symptoms return at some point after you begin to increase your carbohydrate intake, you've increased it too much. Reduce it again. You can experiment with your diet and find the ideal amount of carbohydrate consumption. As your health improves, so should your tolerance for carbohydrates. This is especially true if yeast is a factor.

Hypochlorhydra: If there is an underlying zinc deficiency, supplementation can help. There are hydrochloric acid supplements available in health food stores, but it really is a good idea to consult with a physician who deals in natural health care before trying to treat this on your own.

When I first started practicing, I was told by a doctor in my area who I had a great deal of respect for, that if he was only allowed to treat one system in the body, it would be the digestive system. He said that most other diseases started there. That may be an overstatement, but only a little one. The longer I stay in practice, the truer that statement seems to be.

Allergies

An allergy is an inappropriate response to an innocuous substance. Most people think of an allergic reaction as being sudden and severe. You break out in hives after eating strawberries; you smell ragweed and have a sneezing fit; or your eyes itch and water when you're exposed to dust. Allergic responses, however, are not always so obvious.

Allergic reactions are many and varied. The sudden onset of symptoms is only one way to react. If you are mildly allergic to something, it may take several exposures in a short period of time to evoke a response. For example, a milk allergy may give you sinus problems, but if you only have a little milk during the course of a week, you may not experience any symptoms. If, however, you have a lot of milk on a given day or have milk several days in a row, and your sinuses begin to fill up, you may never make the connection between your symptoms and the allergy.

There is another type of allergic reaction, known as the addictive allergy. This is an allergic reaction where you crave the food that you are allergic to. You crave the substance like an alcoholic craves alcohol. In fact, Theron Randolph, a noted allergist and pioneer in the field of environmental medicine, calls alcoholism the ultimate food allergy.

Dr. Randolph was one of the first, if not the first doctor to espouse the idea of an addictive allergy. He did so in the face of criticism from his colleagues. His contribution to health care and his courage should put his name among the likes of Pasteur in the history of medicine. One of Dr. Randolph's books, *An Alternative Approach to Allergies*, is particularly worth getting. It will cover the topic of allergies in much more depth than these few pages.

People with addictive allergies eat the food that they are addicted to every day. They usually don't even know that they are allergic to that food. In fact, when told that they may be allergic to a favorite food, they are incredulous. "I can't be allergic to *that*, I eat it every day." The real tip-off to an addictive allergy is that the patient is very distressed at the idea of giving up that particular food, much the same way that an alcoholic is distressed at the idea of giving up alcohol.

People with addictive allergies suffer from a wide variety of symptoms, including fatigue, obesity, overeating, chronic sinus problems, repeated infections, hives, rashes, acne or other skin problems, digestive problems, headaches, anxiety depression, joint pain or hypoglycemia. Even gallstones may be caused by allergies. Instead of having sudden and severe symptoms, people with addictive allergies have chronic problems that they seldom associate with their allergy.

138

These are often patients who are just plain sick and go from doctor to doctor and receive little help. Frequently a doctor will tell them that it is all in their head. It is the ultimate medical ego trip, "If I can't fix you, you must be a hypochondriac." Along with all of the physical misery these patients suffer, sometimes they also begin to believe that they are crazy.

There is a link between allergies and digestive problems. One clinical study showed that children with giardiasis (an amoebic parasite), produced more allergic antigens than children who were not infected with the parasite. Leaky gut, which can cause allergies by allowing foreign material into the bloodstream, can be caused by parasites.

Allergic reactions can also cause leaky gut. It's a chicken-and-egg situation. Which came first, the allergy or the digestive problem? Both problems need to be addressed. You need to know what your allergens are, and you need to address any digestive problems that are present.

The concept of addictive allergy is still not widely accepted. Many allergists only believe in immediate allergic reactions. However, when an addictive allergy is identified, and that substance is avoided, the patient often improves dramatically.

Some of the more common foods Americans are allergic to include: corn, dairy, wheat, yeast, eggs, citrus, nightshade vegetables (tomato, pepper, potato), coffee, chocolate and soy. Finding foods that you have addictive allergies to may be tricky.

The lab tests for allergies are far from perfect. The traditional scratch tests are very inaccurate. In fact, according to Dr. Marshal Mandell, they may be as much as 80% inaccurate. Blood tests for allergies are available. The RAST test, which is an acronym for radioallerosorbent test, is a one where the blood is exposed to an allergen and the immune response is noted. There are inaccuracies with RAST testing, and it also does not indicate the severity of the allergic response. This is a standard test performed by most hospital labs.

One test worth mentioning here is the ELISA/ACT test. It does measure the severity of the immune response. It is advanced testing for delayed reactions (often called hidden allergies) to foods and chemicals. It can be done through testing of the body's immune reactive white cells (lymphocytes). ELISA/ACT tests all delayed pathways and can test for reactions to over 300 substances. This test was developed by Dr. Russell Jaffe and is available from Serammune Physician's Labs at 800-553-5472. You can contact their customer service department for more information.

One of the most effective ways of finding allergies is to fast for four days. When you begin eating, introduce only one food each day and watch for a reaction. This approach should be taken only under a doctor's care. You'd be surprised how severely you can react to a food that you used to eat every day, and thought was harmless.

One of the pioneers in the field of food allergy, Dr. Herbert Rinkel, discovered this phenomena quite by accident. Dr. Rinkel and his family ate eggs every day when he was in medical school. His father, a Kansas farmer, sent him a gross of eggs each week to help him hold expenses down.

Dr. Rinkel had a chronic runny nose, and had tried various changes in his diet to get rid of it. He did not consider eggs to be part of his problem because eating large numbers of eggs made no difference in his symptoms. Dr. Rinkel was at a party, and after having no eggs for five days, had a piece of cake. The cake was made with eggs and he immediately collapsed. This is exactly how people with addictive allergies react after removing a substance for several days and then reintroducing it.

Dr. Rinkel's original attitude that the eggs were not part of his problem is the exact attitude most allergists take toward allergy, even today. Eating eggs while in the addictive state makes no changes in the symptoms; therefore, eggs are not the problem. This is the key to the controversy between clinical ecologists, who believe that many, if not most, chronic symptoms can be caused by allergies; and traditional doctors, who believe that allergies result in sudden, definite reactions.

If you suspect that you have food allergies, you could go to a doctor who is recommended by the American Academy of Environmental Medicine. These are doctors who understand the value of natural therapies and are familiar with the concept of addictive allergies. The Academy's number is 303-622-9755.

Treatment for allergies include inoculating small amounts of the antigen (substance that causes the allergy) into the body, or placing a dilute solution of the offending agent under the tongue. Simple avoidance is one approach; you find out what you are allergic to and avoid it. Avoidance becomes difficult if you are allergic to a great many things. Another approach to food allergies is to avoid the substances to which you are allergic and follow the rotary diversified diet, also called the rotation diet. The rotation diet is recommended because eating the same foods over and over again can create new allergies. Sometimes the food can be reintroduced into the diet after a six-week avoidance period. Sometimes patients have so many allergies that total avoidance is impossible. These patients need to follow the rotary diet and avoid the substances to which they react the most.

If you have not identified your food allergies, you can still go on the rotation diet. In fact, it is a way to help your allergies without doing anything that may cause you harm.

During the rotation diet, you may begin to discover which foods upset you. You may become fatigued or feel bloated after a meal containing allergens. You may really miss the allergic food on the three days that you don't eat it. Your pulse may speed up after eating a food that you are allergic to.

Here is a sample of the rotary diversified diet. There is a bigger selection of foods available. This is just a sample to give you an idea how the diet works.

Day	Breakfast	Lunch	Dinner
1	Oatmeal	Avocado, tuna	Turkey, green beans
2	Melon	Pork, cabbage	Halibut, carrots
3	Egg, potato	Lentils	Salmon, rice
4	Berries, yogurt	Swordfish, spinach	Beef, asparagus

In the rotary diet, no food can be eaten more than every four days. Foods in the same family can not be eaten more than every two days. Onion and asparagus are both in the lily family. If you have onion on Monday, you can't have asparagus on Tuesday.

Combination foods are a problem. Mayonnaise, for example, has dairy, eggs, yeast, soy and apple (from cider vinegar). You could not have beef, chicken, strawberries, beans or mushrooms the day after you had mayonnaise. Strawberries are related to apples; beans are related to soy; mushrooms are related to yeast (which is used to ferment the vinegar), chicken is related to egg; and beef is related to dairy.

A partial list of food families is shown below. This is just to give you an idea of some of the relationships. The list is derived from the list in Theron Randolph's book *An Alternative Approach to Allergies*. The list in Dr. Randolph's book was originally printed in "Coping With Your Allergies" by Natalie Golos and Frances Golos Golbitz. These sources will give you a complete listing of the foods and their families.

Fungi: Yeasts and molds, citric acid (a yeast by-product), mushrooms.

Grass: Barley, corn, rice, oat, sugar cane, wheat.

Lily: Aloe, asparagus, chives, garlic, leek, onion.

Goosefoot: Beet, chard, spinach, sugar beet.

Laurel: Avocado, bay leaf, cinnamon, sassafras.

Mustard: Broccoli, Brussel sprouts, cabbage, cauliflower, collards, horseradish, kale, kohlrabi, mustard greens, mustard seed, radish, rutabaga, turnip, watercress.

Rose: Apple, pear, quince, rosehips, almond, apricot, cherry, peach, nectarine, plum, most berries (but not cranberries or blueberries).

Legume: Alfalfa, fava beans, lima beans, mung beans, navy beans, string beans, kidney beans, black-eyed peas, carob, lentil, pea, peanut, soybean.

Carrot: Carrot, anise, caraway, celery, coriander, cumin, dill, fennel, parsley, parsnip.

Mint: Basil, marjoram, oregano, peppermint, rosemary, sage, spearmint, thyme.

Potato: Eggplant, bell peppers, chili peppers, cayenne, paprika, potato, tomato, tobacco.

Composite: Chicory, dandelion, endive, escarole, globe artichoke, Jerusalem artichoke, lettuce, Romaine, safflower oil, sunflower, tarragon.

Gourd: Melons, cucumber, squashes, zucchini.

Bovine: Beef, dairy, buffalo, goat, sheep.

The rotation diet is only one approach to food allergies. People suffering from allergies are not necessarily doomed to a life of avoidance. Since nutritional deficiency contributes to allergies, proper nutritional supplementation can help you to tolerate the things you are sensitive to.

The value of nutritional supplementation in treating allergies is demonstrated by the story of Dr. Stephen Levine. After Dr. Levine received his doctorate, he began working in agricultural biochemistry. He worked with mushrooms, which at a certain stage of their life cycle produce carbon monoxide. Repeated exposure to the carbon monoxide, plus exposure to a variety of chemical solvents and other reagents, undermined Dr. Levine's immune system.

He began to experience frequent adverse reactions to foods. He suffered continually from flu-like symptoms. He had accumulated many allergies. Chemical exposure will do that to you. This is one reason why it is so important to avoid chemical additives, no matter what the "safe" levels are.

Levine became chronically ill and lost much of his motivation to work in the laboratory. He quit his job because any chemical exposure now made him ill. He had extreme fatigue, body aches and nausea. He felt as if he had the flu all of the time.

He went to a clinic, a specially designed ecology unit, which was designed to be chemical and dust-free. Nothing made from plastics or petro chemicals was allowed inside. Only organically grown foods were served. Rooms were specially constructed with walls made of glass and cement blocks. The blocks were painted with special out-gassing paint that was allowed to dry for one year. Floors were made of stone or hard vinyl and were also allowed to age. Ceiling were made of mineral rock and lights were fluorescent with metal fixtures. Mattresses, linens and curtains were all made of cotton and laundered in nondetergent soaps. Heating and air-conditioning were all electric. Special activated charcoal filters were used to eliminate fumes. The rooms were designed so that there was no possible chemical exposure.

Dr. Levine was put on a fast for four days, where he went through severe withdrawal symptoms, a sign of addictive allergy. Allergies are often addictive, and the patient denied the allergen will often suffer an exacerbation of symptoms when the allergen is removed. The patient often suffers like a withdrawing alcoholic or heroin addict. Levine was diagnosed as having many food allergies, along with his chemical sensitivities.

He was given antigen treatments and told to live near the ocean and stay away from all modern conveniences. He moved out of his house and began living in a shed on his property made of wood and concrete. Even living in the absence of chemicals, he felt achiness and flu-like symptoms. Avoidance of the allergens was not successful; it was not an effective therapy.

In an effort to improve his health, Dr. Levine began to experiment with taking vitamins. Magnesium and calcium and vitamins A, B, C and E all helped, but his symptoms always returned. He tried trace minerals and adrenal supplements. In four and a half months he felt stronger. In six months he was able to eat normally. With the vitamin regimen he created for himself, he was able to move back into his house.

Dr. Levine was able to rid himself of his allergic symptoms with vitamin supplementation. Clinically, many doctors who deal in natural health care have noticed that allergies can be eliminated with proper nutrition and vitamin supplementation. Vitamin C helps to prevent the rise of histamine in an allergic response. Various trace minerals help to control allergy symptoms as well.

In his book *Brain Allergies*, Dr. William Philpott has some case histories of patients with mental problems who, by removing food allergens from their diet, experienced great improvement in their psychological symptoms. Many of the patients began to be able to tolerate their allergic foods after vitamin supplementation.

Chiropractic and applied kinesiology techniques, like reflex points and cranial-sacral adjusting, are also helpful to allergy sufferers. Improving the function of the nervous system has a direct effect on the immune system. Many patients notice that their allergies improve after beginning chiropractic or applied kinesiology treatments. Many chiropractors have patients whose allergies improved simply from chiropractic adjustments.

One common allergy is hay fever. It spoils an entire season for many Americans. They spend the spring, fall or both taking antihistamines and feeling drowsy. One very simple thing to do that improves the symptoms of hay fever is to go on a hypoglycemic diet. Simply avoid sugar and refined grains (white rice, white flour), and eat every two hours. The itching eyes of hay fever can be relieved by taking about 10,000 units of vitamin A each day for about a week. Don't take large doses of vitamin A for long periods of time, it can be toxic.

Allergies are more common than most people realize. They are effectively treated by a wide variety of approaches. What works for allergies is the same philosophy that works for many other ailments: Treat the person who has the allergy and not simply treat the allergy. At the end of the book is a healing exercise. If you suffer from allergies, do the exercise every day. The tape set that accompanies this book has a healing exercise that you can listen to daily.

Chemical Exposure

Chemical exposure can cause a wide variety of symptoms, including fatigue, allergies and even cancer. Dr. Levine's case demonstrates the ability of chemicals to seriously undermine anyone's health. Some occupations that involve chemical exposure are farmers, hairdressers, photographers, people working in refineries and factories, people working on or around airplanes, truck drivers, auto mechanics, painters, doctors and x-ray technicians.

Heavy Metals

Megadeath or Van Halen don't have anything to do with health (other than their role in causing a little premature hearing loss). Heavy metals such as lead (without the Zeppelin), cadmium and mercury are deadly poisons. Heavy metal poisoning can occur from pesticides, water pipes, fish and pollution. There has been a high incidence of lead poisoning among people rehabbing old buildings because of the lead in old paint.

Claire Patterson, Ph.D., a geologist at the California Institute of Technology, is of the opinion that we are all subclinically lead poisoned. She postulates that people living today have approximately 1000 times the amount of lead in their bodies as people living 500 years ago. Subclinical lead poisoning is not something most doctors look for when trying to diagnose fatigue.

Cadmium is a heavy metal that is particularly toxic to the immune system. The major source of cadmium is cigarette smoke. It is also used to harden rubber, so it is found in tires and rubber-backed carpets. Incinerators often release cadmium into the air, since the metal is very volatile.

Mercury poisoning may be another source of fatigue. Many dentists engage in the controversial practice of removing mercury amalgam fillings to treat fatigue and immune system problems. There may be value in replacing mercury fillings with other material, since they wear out and have to be replaced anyway. Having all of your fillings removed is painful and expensive and may not be the first thing you would want to do to treat your fatigue. Having your dentist use other materials to replace your mercury fillings as they wear out may be a better approach. Mercury is also found in many large, ocean-going fish. Eating tuna, lobster, swordfish and salmon on a regular basis may cause mercury toxicity in the body.

Aluminum has been linked to Alzheimer's disease, amyotrophic lateral sclerosis (also called ALS or Lou Geherig's disease) and other neurological problems. Aluminum is in most table salt, many antacids and many deodorants.

Detection of heavy metals in the body can be done by testing blood, urine or hair. Hair analysis is still rather controversial, but it is inexpensive and many physicians claim that it is a valuable diagnostic tool.

If heavy metals are found, chelation therapy is very effective at eliminating them. In chelation therapy EDTA (or another chemical, but EDTA is the most commonly used), is injected into the bloodstream. The EDTA binds to metals like lead or mercury and enables it to be eliminated from the bloodstream through the kidneys. EDTA also removes some beneficial minerals like magnesium, zinc, calcium, selenium, and so on. Mineral supplementation may be necessary while undergoing chelation.

One controversial use of chelation is for the improvement of vascular diseases. Many proponents of chelation claim that it can be used to get rid of arterial plaquing in heart patients, improve blood circulation in diabetics and help those with phlebitis and other types of peripheral vascular disease.

Carbon Monoxide

In recent years people have become more aware of the dangers of carbon monoxide poisoning. Carbon monoxide detectors have become common. What makes carbon monoxide so dangerous is the fact that it binds to hemoglobin. It has a greater affinity for hemoglobin than oxygen does. It is fairly common knowledge that carbon monoxide poisoning can cause death, literally suffocating its victims. What few people realize is that low level exposure to it can cause fatigue, dizziness and nausea. There is a simple blood test for the levels of carbon monoxide levels in the blood.

What to Do About Chemicals

This section of the book is not written to cause you to be overly concerned about the amount chemicals in the environment. Worry tends to cause paralysis. You simply need to reduce the amount of chemical exposure that you receive. If you have addressed all of the other health issues in this book and your health is not perfect yet, and if you feel that you still need to have more energy, take some small steps to ensure a minimal amount of chemical exposure in your life.

If you are regularly exposed to chemicals, take steps to minimize your exposure. If your job provides protective clothing, wear it. Make sure that ventilation is adequate. See if there are nontoxic substitutes. Taking trace minerals, vitamin C and other antioxidants may mitigate the damage done by the chemicals.

Everyone is always being exposed to chemicals at some level. Air and water pollution exist everywhere on the planet. The problem is compounded by dumping poisons on lawns so they will be pretty and green, and by using bug sprays, room deodorizers, certain cleaning agents and other chemicals. This is chemical exposure that you can control. Tolerate a few more weeds and have an organic lawn, free of herbicides. Make compost and use it instead of chemical fertilizer. There are many companies that sell household products that are chemical free. Buy organically grown food and meats that are raised without the use of antibiotics or steroids. Look at the chemicals in your life and see which ones you can do without.

If smoke, perfume or other chemicals bother you, or if you can't stand to be around new fabrics, in new cars or around building materials, you may have to take more extreme steps in order to feel better. Create a chemical-free sleeping space. Seal off all heating ducts and make sure that the room is heated or cooled only with electricity. Seal all of the windows and the crack under the door. Don't store your clothes in this room. Have no carpeting or manmade fabrics in the room. A HEPA filter will cut down on indoor air pollution. Use cotton for sheets and window coverings.

The chemical-free sleeping area is a rather extreme step, but necessary for many people. Of course, if you take a lesson from Dr. Levine and get someone to help you find the appropriate nutrient supplementation, chemical sensitivity will be less of a problem.

Thyroid

An underfunctioning thyroid gland can cause fatigue and many other health problems. Thyroid patients, like those suffering with leaky gut, dysbiosis and allergies, are often labeled as hypochondriacs. Some of the symptoms they have are muscle weakness; dry, coarse skin; coldness; diminished sweating; weight gain; constipation; excessive or painful menstruation; nervousness; decreased sex drive; brittle nails; poor memory; emotional instability (often tearful for no reason at all); depression, headaches; or swelling of the face and eyelids.

If you are suffering with any of these symptoms, you can take the Barnes basal temperature test. It's a simple test: You don't even need a No. 2 pencil and you don't even have to mark between the lines. All you need is a mercury thermometer. Before you go to bed at night, shake down the thermometer and have it ready on your night stand. When you wake up in the morning, *before you do anything else*, put the thermometer in your axilla (armpit). Lay in bed, don't do anything for 10 minutes and leave the thermometer there.

Do the test for a few mornings in a row. Your temperature should be between 97.8 and 98.2 degrees Fahrenheit. It is any lower than that, you could have an underfunctioning thyroid.

Many times the test will show a thyroid problem when the laboratory tests are normal. Dr. Broda Barnes in his book *Hypothyroidism: The Unsuspected Illness,* says that the temperature test is much more accurate than the standard blood tests. Of course, if you suspect thyroid problems, you should consult with your doctor. I would much rather have you consult with your doctor than with the law firm of McGreedy, Larsen and Snatch.

Hypothyroidism is especially common in the Midwest, the so-called goiter belt, because of the lack of iodine in the soil. The RDA for iodine is 100 mcg. for women and 120 mcg. for men.

People living in areas near the seashore get much more iodine than people who live inland. Seafood and kelp are very high in iodine. Also, fruits and vegetables grown near the ocean have much more iodine because the iodine content of the soil is much higher than it is inland.

Iodized salt doesn't quite supply the amount of iodine needed by many people. It is, however, enough to cut down on the incidence of one of the symptoms of hypothyroidism: the goiter.

Iodine deficiency isn't the only cause of hypothyroidism. There is a genetic connection. The tendency to have an underfunctioning thyroid runs in families. Members of the same family may be intolerant to even slight decreases in iodine intake.

Another cause of hypothyroidism is pollution. Some chemicals that are in the air and water supply affect the thyroid. Phthalate esters, which are added to plastic to give it flexibility, are toxic to the thyroid. Drinking liquids that are stored in plastic may cause a problem because small amounts of plastic from the container leaches into the liquid. Nitrites, found in processed meats, are toxic to the thyroid and may supperss thyroid function. Also, do you remember sulfamethazine? That's the antibiotic that hog farmers use; it's toxic to the thyroid.

It may be possible to improve your thyroid function without taking any drugs. Taking kelp will help. You can also take a protomorphogen, like the one discussed in the section on adrenal glands. It is the desiccated gland, with the hormone removed.

Other nutrients help thyroid function. The amino acid, tyrosine is very similar in structure to thyroid hormone. Vitamins B, C and E and essential fatty acids are also necessary for proper thyroid function. Essential fatty acids, vitamin A, and vitamin E are not provided in sufficient amounts in today's popular low-fat diets. If strong light bothers your eyes or if you have trouble seeing at night, you may need vitamin A and possibly zinc. Be careful; taking high doses of vitamin A can be toxic. Taking beta carotene, the precursor to vitamin A, is safer. Some individuals, however, have trouble converting beta carotene to vitamin A; thus vitamin A supplementation may be necessary.

A diet consisting of whole foods, such as the caveman diet, is necessary for proper thyroid function. Taking kelp, a good quality multiple vitamin, flax oil, tyrosine and thyroid protomorphogen may help to stimulate the thyroid gland.

Of course, diagnosing and treating your own thyroid problem will put you in the same category as Mr. Needlebrain. If you take your basal body temperature and it is low, find a physician who understands natural health care to help you with this. If the nutritional approach doesn't work, you may need a prescription for thyroid medication.

Structural Problems—Bodywork

Ninety-eight percent of all Americans will have back pain at some point in their lives. Some of the causes of back pain are muscle imbalance, poor body mechanics, being overweight, lack of exercise, poor footwear (especially high heels), poor posture, stress and even smoking. All these can predispose you to back pain.

People in jobs that are sedentary, that involve working on computers or being on the phone are usually prone to back and neck pain. Such jobs are usually more fatiguing than jobs that involve physical activity. Proper ergonomics, good posture, taking time to stretch and getting plenty of physical exercise will go a long way to minimize the aches and pains of having a desk job.

Often it is necessary to get outside help with your structural problems. Chiropractic, massage, Rolfing and other types of bodywork will help you to feel better and have more energy. Chiropractic is an excellent way to improve posture and reduce structural stress. A chiropractor manipulates or "adjusts" the spine to relieve pressure on spinal nerves. This relieves pain, reduces muscle spasm and improves general health.

Pain and muscle spasm are fatiguing, as anyone who has had chronic pain can attest. The body doesn't know the difference between muscle spasm and a muscle that is constantly working. Drugs mask the symptoms, but don't solve the problem.

Anti-inflammatory drugs cause intestinal bleeding and leaky gut. Many of these drugs interfere with normal fat metabolism and prostaglandin synthesis. Acetomenaphin is very hard on your kidneys and liver. Chiropractic and other forms of hands on health care control pain without the use of drugs. Along with relief from headaches, neck and back pain and muscle spasm, chiropractic adjustments improve the function of the nervous system. They help the body to heal itself and to keep itself healthy.

Many people think of chiropractors as bone doctors, but in reality, they work with the nervous system. **Chiropractic's effect on the nervous system extends to the autonomic nervous system and to**

the organs. Chiropractic care and other types of bodywork relieve stress, improve health and increase energy. Lifelong chiropractic patients can attest to this.

One major cause of pain, headaches, muscle spasms and many other symptoms is the temporomandibular or TMJ (jaw joint). Many people suffering with chronic pain and unable to get help have problems with their jaw joint. The TMJ is a balancing organ, much like the inner ear. It can literally affect any part of the body.

In neurology texts you will see a homunculus, which is Latin for "little man." A homunculus is the brain's representation of the body. The picture representing the homunculus is a man with a great big face, big hands, big feet and a little tiny body. The picture is drawn proportionally to show how much of the brain is devoted to running each area of the body. Certain areas of the body require more brain tissue to control them than do other parts of the body. For example, there is more sensitivity and movement in the hands than there is in the buttocks. In order for that to be possible, a larger portion of the brain is devoted to controlling the hands than the buttocks. (This is true for the entire population, with the possible exception of this dancer I saw in LA.)

A very large portion of your brain is devoted to the TMJ. In fact, more of the brain is involved with TMJ function than with any other joint in the body. This is a very important fact when it comes to posture, muscle spasm and pain.

Your body has priorities when it comes to posture. For instance, keeping your eyes level is one of your body's priorities. It is done automatically, and, if necessary, at the expense of any other postural consideration. For instance, if someone has a short leg, the head will tilt or the spine will curve so that the difference between the leg lengths will not affect the eyes being level. Try to spend the day with your head tilted and your eyes unlevel. You will get a terrific headache.

The body has a similar priority with the TMJ. It wants to keep the jaw level. Since so much brain tissue is devoted to balancing the jaw, if there is a little bit of spasm in one of the jaw muscles or if the jaw does not hang normally, the body will arrange its posture around the jaw.

From your body's point of view, having the head or shoulders tilted, neck rotated and even hips out of balance is much less of a problem than to have the jaw hang crookedly. The body will arrange itself as best it can to keep the eyes and jaw level. This fact sometimes makes it difficult to correct some postural problems.

For many people with TMJ syndrome, this results in pain, especially in the neck and upper back, muscle spasm, fatigue or headaches. Some patients even experience low back pain, sciatica or digestive disturbance.

If you clench your jaw, grind your teeth at night, have trouble with occlusion (how your teeth fit) or if your jaw clicks, you may be having trouble with your TMJ. It is, however, possible to have TMJ syndrome and not notice any problem with your jaw. There are some ways to tell if TMJ may be a problem. If you take the three middle fingers of your dominant hand and bend them, the three knuckles of your proximal interphalangial joint (that's just the finger joint that's closest to the hand, but not the one that connects the fingers to the hand) should fit into your mouth. Another possible indication of a TMJ problem is a jaw that wobbles when you open it slowly. Look in the mirror and slowly open your jaw. It should open straight, with no deviations from side to side.

Treatment for TMJ syndrome can be anything from applied kinesiology, muscle balancing and chiropractic adjustments, to a bite guard, to braces. It all depends on the severity of the problem and its cause. Bruxing, or grinding of the teeth, can be caused by a filling being too high, malocclusion (teeth not fitting properly together), imbalance of the TMJ muscles, stress or even food allergies.

Bruxing, if it persists can damage the teeth or the temperomandibular joint itself, and may make the use of dental appliances necessary. Dentists use bite guards or braces to change how the upper and lower teeth fit together. This will change the alignment of the jaw, relaxing the TMJ muscles. If the joint is severely damaged from bruxing or actual trauma, surgery is sometimes recommended. This is an extreme measure, and should be a last resort.

Chiropractors, applied kinesiologists, Rolfers and cranio-sacral therapists work directly on the jaw joint, the muscles, the cervical spine and on cranial bones to try to achieve the same result. Sometimes a combination of dental and other therapies is effective.

Cranial adjusting and cranio-sacral therapy have been mentioned in several places in this text. This is a very important therapy for people with allergies, TMJ, chemical toxicity and other problems. The brain fag discussed by doctors who work with clinical ecology can be addressed by cranial adjusting.

Most people, including many physicians, think of the skull as a fixed, immovable bone. In reality, the skull consists of 22 bones that move very slightly. The bones are connected by joints called sutures. Not only are the bones of the skull able to move, they must move in a very specific fashion for you to enjoy good health.

If you look at the way the gills of a fish move, you have an idea of how your skull moves. The human skull moves a bit less that the gills of a fish. This motion, however small, must be present and normal, or you may suffer from headaches, dizziness or fatigue.

People suffering from brain fag or deep fatigue, which many of them describe as being like a hangover, usually have improper cranial motion. They respond very well to cranial adjusting. Very often a patient who has a treatment that addresses cranial motion will use the phrase, "I feel like my lights are back on!"

Not only does the correction of cranial faults make you feel better, it helps your nervous system overcome many health problems. Cranial adjusting improves nervous system function, much the same way that chiropractic does.

Chronic Fatigue Syndrome

The symptoms of chronic fatigue syndrome (CFS) are so many and varied that some doctors don't even believe that it exists. Many view it as hypochondria or as a manifestation of depression. The estimated three million CFS sufferers in the United States may have any of the following symptoms: fatigue, poor concentration, sleep disturbances, headaches, low-grade afternoon fever, swollen lymph glands, sore throat, depression, muscle aches, joint pain, mental confusion, anxiety attacks, weight loss or skin rashes.

The one symptom all CFS sufferers have is a profound fatigue that does not seem to be relieved by sleep. The fatigue and symptoms are so severe that approximately half of all CFS patients cannot work and a quarter of them are bedridden. Symptoms last for a few months to two years or more, with one-third of the patients being sick for more than two years.

Part of the confusion the medical community has with defining CFS stems from several facts. In the mid-1980s the medical literature tried to define CFS as a chronic infection caused by Epstein-Barr virus (a distant relative of Roseanne). The problem is that not all of the patients suffering with the symptoms of chronic fatigue syndrome have the Epstein-Barr virus.

Since the time of Pasteur, most diseases have been defined as having a single infectious agent. Medicine seems to be obsessed with the idea of a single microorganism causing disease. If some CFS sufferers have Epstein-Barr, and others do not, it is taken as proof that CFS is not a distinct disease entity.

What happens in CFS is much more complex than a simple viral infection. Many of the things we've already discussed may be involved in chronic fatigue syndrome. Consider the case of Dr. Stephen Levine. His symptoms could classify him as a CSF patient. He had profound fatigue, weakness and joint pain. The cause of his problem was chemical exposure and multiple allergies.

Often many infectious agents are involved. There may be yeast or parasitic infestation of the bowel, as well as a viral infection. There may be viruses other than Epstein-Barr. Cytomegalovirus and a virus in the Herpes family have also been implicated in CFS.

The symptoms of allergies, candidiasis, chemical exposure, heavy metals, thyroid problems and parasites can all be interpreted as CFS. Poor diet, chemical exposure, poor digestion and infectious agents are all like straw on the camel's back. If there are enough assaults on the immune system and it breaks down, you have chronic fatigue syndrome.

An effective approach to CFS is just a matter of breaking it down into components and treating each individual problem. Parasites and yeast should be tested for and treated. Antibodies for Epstein-Barr, Herpes and Cytomegalovirus should be tested for. Leaky gut can be tested for by taking the intestinal permeability test. Testing for heavy metals is also a good idea.

If Epstein-Barr or other virus is present, there are a number of natural antiviral substances that can be taken. These include vitamin C, quercetin, blue-green algae, St. John's wort, lysine, lepotania and monolauric acid. Standard Process makes a product called Congaplex which is a very good combination of substances that fight viruses and enhance immunity.

As Dr. Levine discovered in his own case, there are several nutrients that can be taken to enhance immunity. Vitamin A, B6, coenzyme Q-10, vitamin C, trace minerals and antioxidants all help the immunity. Herbs like echinacea and astragalus also stimulate the immune system.

A variety of vitamins and herbs have been given to improve mental function and increase energy. Vitamin B complex, choline, glutathione, ginseng and ginkgo biloba are examples of these substances. It must be stressed that each individual is different, and there is no single CFS nutritional regimen. Patients will respond most to the nutrients they are most deficient in or the ones that directly address their unique biochemical problems.

Treatment of digestive problems, dysbiosis and leaky gut, as discussed in other sections, can be very important to CFS patients. Chelation, although controversial, may be beneficial to those suffering from heavy metal poisoning. Many people have immediate relief from their fatigue after undergoing chelation therapy.

Good nutrition and avoiding chemical additives and other toxins are vital to a return to good health. In fact, it can be argued that chemicals and lack of nutrients in food are contributing factors to CFS, allergies and poor health in general.

Some medical doctors use certain drugs with some of their CFS patients. Histamine blockers and antiviral drugs are sometimes used as well as antifungal and antiparasitic drugs. Other doctors try very hard not to use drugs and try to find herbal and nutritional alternatives because the natural substances are much less stressful to the body.

As you can see, diagnosing and treating CFS is very complex and something that you may not want to undertake on your own. Otherwise you may end up following some ill-conceived, hit-or-miss, blending of nutritional and herbal therapies that may not work. I see this in my office all of the time. People come in complaining of fatigue and they also have a shoulder problem caused by lugging around a 50-pound bag full of vitamins and herbs. They've tried every panacea offered up by every expert, with only marginal results.

The way to treat CFS is to follow a good basic nutritional and health plan, like the one offered in the first part of this book. Follow all components of the 30-day plan. I know it sounds prejudiced, but a good chiropractor/applied kinesiologist can work wonders. Diagnostic tests must be performed to find dysbiosis, leaky gut, allergies and heavy metals. Appropriate nutritional supplementation and herbal therapies must be implemented. One very valuable thing you can do for yourself is to do the healing exercise at the end of this book. You may find it easier to use the healing tape; it is a powerful tool. Listen to it on a regular basis.

Now What?

For most people, following the 30-day plan in the first part of the book and doing the exercises will give them incredible energy. Simply returning to healthy habits and using your mind to focus on having energy will work miracles. If you ever saw the movie The Karate Kid, you'll remember that the character played by Ralph Moccaicio prepared for the tournament at the end of the movie by learning four very basic moves, but he did them flawlessly. The four basic moves to having energy is to get optimum food, air, water and thought.

Consider the two lunches listed earlier in the book. The nutritional difference between them is phenomenal. The lunch with the turkey on whole wheat had six times as much folic acid, and that's only one nutrient. Look at how taking extra nutrients solved Dr. Levine's health problem. Every day, each decision that you make about your food either moves you toward health or away from it. On a daily basis, eating nutrient-rich, chemical-free food will make a tremendous difference in how you feel. It's simple, like "wax on, wax off," but it works.

Every part of the 30-day plan is important in giving you boundless energy. The breathing and mental exercises are especially important. Your mind is a powerful tool. Use it to get the results you desire.

Even with following the 30-day plan, some will still see room for improvement in their health. The second part of this book was designed to teach you about some common causes of fatigue. Not every health problem that causes fatigue was covered; that would turn this into a ponderous medical text. The health topics covered in the second part are things that are likely to be missed in a traditional medical examination.

This book is not meant to be an indictment of the medical profession, as so many books about natural health care are. We see so many diatribes about evil doctors conspiring to treat us with drugs and suppress natural remedies. That probably isn't the case. It's just that modern medicine is very conservative and very crisis oriented, but that's not all bad.

How would you like to get hit by a train and as they are wheeling you into the ER, have the doctor recommend moxibustion and aroma therapy? You would probably rather he or she ordered x-rays and MRIs, all that traditional, conservative stuff. You'd probably be very glad that drugs to control your pain were available. Not very holistic, but very effective.

Some of the topics covered in the second part of this book are controversial and may not be well received by many doctors. However, if you have health problems and have not been helped by traditional medicine, it gives you somewhere else to look for help.

If you suspect that allergies are a problem for you, take some time to learn about them. Get yourself a copy of *An Alternative Approach to Allergies* by Theron Randolph. *Brain Allergies* by William Philpott, M.D. and *Dr. Mandell's Five-Day Allergy Relief System* by Marshal Mandell, M.D. are also very good. Don't just read about allergies and try to treat yourself. You can get a physician referral from the American Academy of Environmental Medicine. The phone number is 303-622-9755. Dr. Russell Jaffe is the inventor of the ELISA/ACT test. You can get a physician referral from his company, Serammune Physicians Lab at 800-553-5472.

If you have problems with digestion or dysbiosis, you can get a physician referral from Meridian Valley Clinical Laboratory at 800-234-6825 or Great Smokies Diagnostic Laboratory at 800-522-4762. This way you can find a physician who uses stool analysis to diagnose digestive problems. Meridian Valley also does allergy testing, hair analysis and various blood tests.

If you suspect that candida is a problem, you may want to read Dr. William Crook's book *The Yeast Connection*. Don't try to diagnose and treat yourself from the book. In general, that's not a good idea. Also, there is a wide variety of approaches to candidiasis. Dr. Crook's book does provide a good explanation of candida and will enrich your understanding of candidiasis.

If you have Crohn's disease, ulcerative colitis, cystic fibrosis of the pancreas, celiac disease or chronic diarrhea, get a copy of Elaine Gottschall's book *Food and the Gut Reaction*. Of course discuss the book with your physician before changing your diet. Again, this can't be stressed enough; don't diagnose and treat yourself.

To read more about thyroid, get a copy of Dr. Broda Barnes' book *Thyroid: the Undiagnosed Illness*. Do this especially if your morning axillary temperature is below 97.8 degrees Fahrenheit. There is another book on thyroid by Stephen Langer, M.D. and James F. Scheer, with the unassuming title of *Solved: The Riddle of Illness*.

If you haven't already done so, give chiropractic a try. You will be amazed at what regular chiropractic adjustments can do for the state of your health. The International College of Applied Kinesiology is a good place to get a referral for a chiropractor. The number is 913-542-1801.

The road to good health is always under repair. Maintain your health and you will be rewarded with plenty of energy and a sense of well-being.

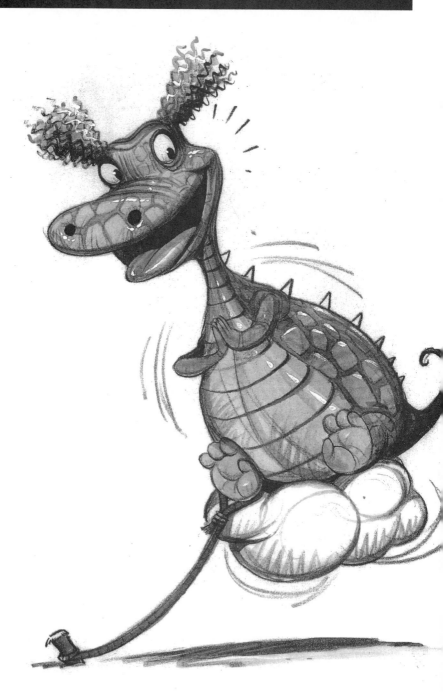

These exercises use the concepts of NLP, hypnosis and meditation. NLP is an acronym for Neuro Linguistic Programming, which is a body of knowledge for being able to duplicate or model excellence and for accelerated learning. It was developed by Richard Bandler and John Grinder in the 1970s.

NLP is the study of how we humans process information and how it affects our behavior. **The word neuro refers to the nervous system.** It is really simple—it's about how your brain works, your thinking processes and the five senses of sight, sound, feelings, smell and taste. In NLP the senses are referred to as the modalities of visual, auditory, kinesthetic, olfactory and gustatory.

Linguistic refers to our language, how we use it and are influenced by it. This includes our nonverbal communications as well. Language is the means through which our neural representations are ordered and given meaning.

Programming refers to our ability to organize our communication and neurology to accomplish specific goals, results and direction in our lives. We can control our neurology and our communication.

Simply put, our words and pictures create our feelings and behaviors. Our behaviors and our experiences have structure. Once we learn how we can reorder the information on how feelings are made and the strategies for creating good feelings, we can get rid of old beliefs that limited you in the past and build new powerful, positive beliefs to enrich our lives—to create for yourself your desires, hopes and dreams.

In the exercises in the book, more so in the tapes, we will be using visualization, anchoring, physiology and directing your focus by learning to ask better questions. The exercises and tapes will help you to create new neural pathways in your brain and a healthier body and soul. At the end of this section we will tell you how you can get the tapes if you choose to use them.

All of these exercises will require you to visualize. Many people don't believe that they visualize, and they do. Everyone visualizes. Just because you don't see bright, Technicolor pictures that look like they were created by Steven Spielberg, doesn't mean that you don't visualize. Try not to see a purple gorilla. See, your mind formed some sort of image. How do you know where you parked your car or what color your living room is? You know because you formed a mental picture; you visualized them. You can't help it; your mind creates pictures all of the time. Visualization is merely the art of deciding what those pictures will be.

In fact, whenever you are to create an image in one of the exercises, do it with full sensory acuity or awareness. That is to say create the image vividly, using all of the senses. See the sights, hear the sounds and feel the feelings. Your mind is very powerful, and it will create what you desire more effectively when you involve all of the senses; in other words, when it is sensory-based.

Our purpose and our intent for providing you with the following exercises in the book is to help yourself to assist you to create for yourself your compelling future. To create for yourself now and in the present incredible health and excellent energy. So we well take you through these exercises, step by step.

Exercise #1: Habit change.

Purpose: To eliminate an old, undesired behavior.

Beginning now with the first exercise that can be used to change an old habit. For just a moment, picture in your mind a habit that you want now to eliminate. Make it a large, bright picture of yourself just before, or as you are beginning to indulge in that undesired habit.

Take that picture for just a moment and set it aside. Now, create another picture. Create a picture of the desired habit or behavior that you choose to have and, as you see yourself, with total energy, feeling rested, relaxed and stress-free. Feel the way you want to feel. Look the way you want to look. See yourself in control of your own destiny. Make the image contain all of the good things you will have, once you eliminate that old habit. Will you lose weight? Will you look better? Will you have more energy? Vividly imagine yourself the way you want to be. What is it like to be in control of all of the choices in your life? Make this image completely compelling to you. Whatever it takes. You can make it bright or you can make it bigger. If there is sound, make the sound a compelling sound. A sound that will motivate you to create this change now and to eliminate the old, unwanted behavior perhaps. A voice telling you what this will give you when you replace the old behavior with the new, better one. That's right; very good. Now, set that picture aside for just a moment.

Look at that large, bright image of the old behavior. Take your desired image, your desired state, that behavior that you really want to have and place that as a tiny dark image in the lower left-hand corner of that picture.

What you do next is very quick, because the brain works very quickly. And the brain wants this done fast. Have the large, bright picture of the old behavior to get suddenly dark. Have the small picture to just spring up, to become very huge, very bright, very big and to spring up and replace that old picture, very quickly as it shatters the old picture into a million pieces. Do this process very quickly. Do it five times in a row, and each time you do it, you can make the sound, "yes." Each time you do it, open your eyes briefly for one second. Close your eyes and do it again. Do it rapidly. Do it five times in a row.

In this exercise, as you look at the pictures, the brain is saying, "Not this," (to the old picture); "this" (to the new picture). You will notice that the big, bright image of your desired behavior is compelling, you feel good, it is more real and more achievable. You can do it.

Exercise #2: Habit change. Installing a good habit.

Purpose: To install your new desired behavior.

Create a picture of yourself, the way that you choose to be now. Make it a picture that you really, really desire. Visualize yourself in excellent physical condition with plenty of energy. Looking good, feeling good, whatever that means to you. Create in your mind an ideal version of yourself. How will it be when you have complete control in all aspects of your life? How do you really want to be? Create the burning desire, vividly in your mind. What do you really want your life to be like?

Have this excellent vision of yourself doing whatever or performing whatever you wish to perform, exercising whatever habits you wish to perform. For example: eating vegetables, exercising, eating nutritious, healthy food, drinking water. These are all examples of the types of habits that you may want or want to visualize yourself doing since they create good health.

Take the image of the perfect image of yourself performing the desired habit. Now really create it. A compelling, wonderful image. Imagine that picture being pulled back as if it were in a slingshot. Just pulling it back, pulling it back, pulling it back. Farther away, getting smaller and smaller. Being pulled back by a slingshot. And when it is so far away that it's a tiny dot, release it from the sling shot, as if it were fired from the slingshot and notice the power and the speed with which that picture moves toward you. Inside, notice how it feels now that you've installed this picture inside your brain and now that you've installed this behavior inside yourself.

Exercise #3: Sleeping.

Purpose: To enable you to sleep well through the night.

Set the direction for your mind in this manner: "I would like my unconscious mind to experience with pictures, sounds and feelings the benefits of being able to fall asleep easily and sleep deeply, continuously and through all the night and to awaken me at {whatever time you choose to awaken}"

Now the reason we say review with pictures, sounds and feelings is because this is a sensory-based experience. When you use your senses of sight, hearing and feeling; experience it fully, then it becomes more powerful.

Now as you lie in bed at night, what we want you to do is to repeat to yourself three visual statements (pictures), three auditory statements (sounds), and three kinesthetic statements (feelings). Note the following examples, but please use your own sensory experience in your room, as you go to sleep.

Examples of visual statements are: Now I am aware that I see the light. Now I am aware that I see the window. Now I am aware that I see the dresser. These are only examples, you can use these or any other sights that you choose.

Examples of auditory statements are: Now I am aware that I hear my slow, rhythmic breathing. Now I am aware that I hear my heart beat. Now I am aware that I hear the hum of the furnace (or air-conditioning). These are only examples, use any three sounds that you choose.

Examples of kinesthetic statements are: Now I am aware that I feel my toes. Now I am aware that I feel my body between the sheets. Now I am aware that I feel my head resting comfortably on the pillow. Again, these are just examples.

After you do the three visual statements, three auditory statements and three kinesthetic statements, using your own sensory experience to notice each thing, repeat two of each of the statements. Make two visual statements, two auditory statements and two kinesthetic statements.

After you finish making two statements, visual, auditory and kinesthetic, make one statement for each modality, before you fall asleep. Make one visual statement, one auditory statement and one kinesthetic statement, using your own sensory experience. Notice each thing, before you go to sleep.

Now I don't know just how quickly you will fall asleep easily and effortlessly, whether you will fall asleep deeply before you finish the statements or afterwards and you can just close your eyes and pretend to be asleep and you will be.

Exercise #4: Changing your mood or frame of mind.

Purpose: To be able to create any desired emotion, frame of mind or feeling.

We cannot control others and cannot always control our environment, but you can control how you feel. Three ways that you can be in control of your emotions or state of mind are anchors, physiology and questions. The purpose of this exercise is to enable you to create anchors which will give you the tools and resources to change your state of mind and to choose the emotion that you desire to experience. In the tape set we will review anchors and will also teach you how to use your physiology and how to ask powerful questions to create any state of mind you desire.

Anchors involve stimulus-response. For example, do you recall a time when you walked into a room, smelled a fragrance that took you back in time? A very special time? A very special feeling? A special experience? One that I find very powerful for me is to walk into a classroom, smelling the crayons, and the smell of the paste which takes me back to the happy, carefree time when I was in school. Perhaps you have at a point in time had a friendship or a special relationship and you had a favorite song that became an anchor for you. and every time you hear the song, you think of that person. So the song is an anchor, the feeling you get is the emotion, feeling or the state of mind.

A famous example of an anchor, or stimulus-response is Ivan Pavlov's experiment with the dog. Pavlov rang a bell each time he fed the dog. Over a period of time, the dog began to associate the bell with the arrival of food. The bell was an anchor. It was such a powerful anchor that the dog salivated when he heard the bell, even when no food arrived. The bell was the stimulus, salivating was the response.

What we want you to do here is to learn how to use this in a systematic way, to create states, emotions and feelings that you want to feel when you choose to feel them. You will be able to create these feelings instantly.

Remember a specific time when you felt confidence and/or can you fully associate to the confidence. Breathe the way you breathe when you are totally confident, stand the way you stand when you are totally confident. Say what you say to yourself when you are totally confident. Double those feelings. Triple those feelings. Use your senses of sight, sound and feeling to recreate that confidence. When you are totally, completely in a state of confidence, make a fist with your right hand, squeezing it tight. Relax for a moment.

Now, create in yourself a feeling of passion. Remember a time when you felt passionate. You had the intense feeling of caring, of loving what you were doing, of joy; a feeling of passion. Feel what you were feeling at that time. See what you were seeing. Hear what you were hearing. Stand the way you stand when you are totally passionate. Breathe the way you breathe when you are totally passionate. Say what you say to yourself when you are totally passionate. Double those feelings. Intensify those feelings. When you are totally, intensely in a state of passion, make a fist with your right hand. Make it the same way as you made the fist is the first part of the exercise, squeezing it tight. Relax for a moment.

Now, create in yourself a feeling of exhilaration. Remember a time when you felt exhilarated. You had the intense feeling of excitement, happiness, of thrilling anticipation; a feeling of exhilaration. Feel what you were feeling at that time. See what you were seeing. Hear what you were hearing. Stand the way you stand when you are totally exhilarated. Breathe the way you breathe when you are totally exhilarated. Say what you say to yourself when you are totally exhilarated. Double those feelings. Make them stronger! Stronger! When you are totally, intensely in a state of exhilaration, make a fist with your right hand. Make it the same way as you made the fist is the first part of the exercise, squeezing it tight. Relax for a moment.

You have just created an anchor. Whenever you want to experience those intense and positive emotions, all you have to do is to make a fist in exactly the same way as you did during the exercise. You will feel confident, passionate and exhilarated in an instant.

In the tapes we will take you through the steps of anchoring; changing physiology; questions; refocusing on your outcome and direction and creating what you want in your life.

Exercise #5: Reducing stress and creating energy.

Purpose: To ground, center and balance yourself and to focus on your desire to have excellent energy and to feel stress free.

First begin breathing in a relaxed manner. Take the time to really relax. Notice your breathing, your chest rising as you fill your lungs with air. Feel them lower as you exhale. Relax each muscle group, one at a time. Start with your feet, feeling them really relax. The feeling of relaxation moves up your legs. Notice your pelvis and abdomen relax. Feel the muscles letting go as the relaxation spreads to your chest and arms. Experience now your neck muscles, jaw muscles and finally your facial muscles becoming totally relaxed. Find yourself in a comfortable place, close your eyes and then begin to visualize, coming from your spine, a cord attached to your spine and going to the center of the earth and then you might also visualize roots coming from your feet and as you begin to feel balanced, centered grounded.

Next notice if there's any negative energy, any frantic energy, and feelings of tiredness that you might have had before and you can to begin to dump those down that grounding cord and you can make the cord as big as a sewer pipe, if you'd like to. Just dump that down the grounding cord and clear out all of that negative energy, any energy that is less than positive for you and allow it to enter into the earth's energy where it becomes neutralized.

Just imagine that if you have any scattered energy, or any scattered parts of yourself, and begin to focus on bringing those energies, all your own energy back into your own body.

Imagine, above your head is a beautiful blue sky with a brilliant, golden sun and to have that golden, healing energy, that calming energy to begin to enter into your body and if there are any parts of your body that might need special attention, or special healing, send an extra special amount of gold to those parts of your body. Very good. Notice how you feel, centered and balanced, with more energy than before and as you're doing this, inside your mind, create for yourself a picture. A picture of something your really, really want. At this point, since we're talking about health and energy it might be a good idea to use the exercise for health and energy. Notice if there is anything that stands between you and what it is that you really want. Take whatever energy that is and dump that energy down the grounding cord. Allow it to go down the cord, dissolve into the earth's energy and neutralize and as it goes away and you clear that out of your space, out of your energy. Make the picture exactly the way you want to be and as you look at the picture, bring it in closer; to make it brighter you might even want to add color to it if you choose. Look at that picture again, notice how much more attainable it is. Experience how good it makes you feel. And really get into those feelings. Embrace those feelings. Amplify those feelings and make them even bigger. Notice now how good it looks and how much better you feel. And you can continue to focus on that desire and on that goal. Hear what you hear, and make it in surround-sound, really compelling sound, compelling picture and powerful and intense. Now slowly, taking all the time you need, begin to come out at your own rate and speed, whatever is appropriate to you. Come back into the present. Open your eyes with a sense of excellent energy and focus and feeling much better than before, with a beautiful sense of well-being.

Exercise #6: Healing Exercise.

Purpose: To access your unconscious mind's ability to heal and facilitate the healing process. Work with your doctor and use every resource available to you. This is just another resource.

A) Choose what you want to heal.

B) Ask yourself, "How will I know it is healing? What evidence do I need that it is healed?

C) Remember a time when you healed automatically, easily, quickly, like a cut or scrape.

D) Since we store things spatially, notice where you see the image of the illness (in front of you , left, right, down etc.) that you want to heal now. Is it a movie or a still picture? Is it in color or in black and white? Is it large or small? Is it bordered or not. Note all characteristics of the illness including what you may hear.

E) Do the same thing with the healing experience from step C. Notice where the healing is. Is it a movie or a still picture? Is it in color or in black and white? Is it large or small? Is it bordered or not? Note all characteristics of the healing, including what you may hear.

F) Change the illness or unhealed experience to the automatic, easily healed experience by making pictures, sounds and feelings exactly like the healed experience. Put it in the same space as the healed experience and change all aspects of the image to that of the healed experience. For example: If you visualize the time you healed easily as a small, black and white picture and the vision of the illness is a large, bright, color picture, change the image of the illness to a small, black and white picture. Change all aspects of the image, including where it is.

G) Ask all parts of yourself if they will see the benefits to yourself and others of allowing this healing to take place. Also ask your unconscious mind to support you by continuing the healing process and moving forward in the direction of excellent health.

The Tapes

When you use the tapes with the exercises, we'll literally take you through the entire process. We will guide you through the exercises and the meditations and we will make this journey with you. These tapes can be used as often as you like. You can use them to reach goals that you choose to reach. So this is in the interest of serving you and just being tour guides to assist you through the wonderful adventure of your own mind and how to create mind-body wellness.

If you would like a copy of the tapes, call 800-672-2250.

Achlorhydra: Absence of stomach acid.

Amino acid: An organic molecule that has both an amino (NH2) and a carboxyl (COOH) group. The basic formula is NH2-R-COOH. Amino acids are the building blocks of which proteins are constructed.

Antioxidant: Nutrients that protect the body against free radicals. These include vitamin C, vitamin E, beta carotene and selenium.

Applied kinesiology: System of muscle testing and balancing for diagnosis and treatment. Used by chiropractors and other health care practitioners.

176

Candidiasis: An overabundance of yeast in the bowel.

Carbohydrate: A group of chemical substances, including sugars, glycogen, starches, dextrins and cellulose that contain only carbon, oxygen and hydrogen. One of the three major classes of food, which include carbohydrate, fat and protein. Carbohydrates include sugars, which are simple six-carbon molecules called monsaccharides or twelve-carbon molecules which are known as disaccharides. Polysaccharides are long molecules. They are either starches or glycogen. Sugars, starches and glycogen are used by the body as fuel. Sources of carbohydrate in food are: fruit, potatoes, beans, corn, rice, wheat and other grains.

Chiropractic: A holistic and natural healing art that is centered around balancing vertebrae that are out of alignment. A chiropractor works with vertebrae because they affect the nervous system. By working with the nervous system, all aspects of health can be affected. Chiro is from the Egyptian word meaning hand. It was created in1895 by D.D. Palmer in its present form, but vertebral alignment has been used as a therapy since ancient times. Today chiropractors use many forms of therapy, but do not prescribe drugs or perform surgery.

Dysbiosis: This is a condition where there is improper flora in the bowel. It can refer to the overgrowth of yeast, pathologic bacteria or parasites. It can also refer to an absence of normal flora or bacteria that are present in an area of the digestive tract that normally doesn't have bacteria.

Essential amino acid: These are amino acids that must be supplied by the diet. The body cannot produce them from other amino acids. These include: histidine, isoleucine, leucine, methionine, phenylalanine, threonine, tryptophan and valine.

Essential fatty acid: There are three fatty acids that are considered to be essential. Linoleic, linolenic and arachidonic acids. Although, only linoleic acid is the only unsaturated fatty acid that must be supplied by the diet.

Fascia: A sheet or band of fibrous tissue such as lies deep to the skin, or forms an investment for muscles and various organs of the body. It's connective tissue. It's similar to the material that ligaments and tendons are made of. If you look at a steak and see the white film-like membrane that covers the meat, that's fascia.

Hypochlorhydra: Underproduction of hydrochloric acid by the stomach.

Korsakoff's psychosis: Alcoholic psychosis. It is believed to be a chronic form of Wernike's syndrome. Disorientation, susceptibility to external suggestion and stimulation, amnesia, hallucinations and polyneuritis are some of the symptoms. Also called chronic alcoholic delirium.

Leaky gut: A situation where intestinal permeability is increased and large molecules, which normally would be kept out of the bloodstream, are absorbed. It can be the cause of allergies and autoimmune diseases.

Megaloblastic anemia: An anemia characterized by the presence of large, immature red blood cells. Sometimes seen in severe vitamin B12 deficiency.

Neuro Linguistic Programming: Created by Richard Bandler and John Grinder in the 1970s, it is a study of how the mind works. Neuro refers to the brain and nervous system. Linguistic refers to language and communication, both verbal and nonverbal. Programming refers to the idea that you can control your nervous system and communications (both with yourself and others) to create change in your life, attain goals and create the kind of life that you would like.

NSAID: Nonsteroidal anti-inflammatory drug. Pain medication including drugs like aspirin, Motrin, Advil and Aleve, which also fight inflammation.

Peptide: A small molecule consisting of two or more amino acids. A constituent part of protein.

Protein: Proteins are the principle constituents of the protoplasm of all cells. Large molecules consist of sequences of amino acids. Each protein has a unique, genetically defined amino acid sequence that determines its shape and function. Proteins serve as enzymes, structural elements, hormones or immunoglobulins.

Road apple: Hardened horse turd.

Starch: Any of a group of polysaccharides of the general formula (C6-H10-05) composed of a long chain of glucose. In other words, a long chain of sugar molecules. Starch is the chief storage form of energy in plants. Plants that are high in starch include corn, wheat, rice and potatoes.

Sterol: Steroids with long aliphatic side chains and at least one alcoholic side group. They are fat-soluble. Examples are cholesterol and ergosterol.

Wernike's syndrome: An inflammatory form of encephalopathy caused by a thiamine deficiency with chronic alcoholism as a contributing factor. It is characterized by paralysis of the eye muscles, diplopia, nystagmus, ataxia and mental changes ranging from deterioration and forgetfulness to delirium tremens.

Barnes, Broda. Hypothyroidism: The Unsuspected Illness.

Crook, William. The Yeast Connection.

Gottschall, Elaine. Food and the Gut Reaction.

Hall, Ross Hume. Food for Naught.

Hamilton, Kirk. "Clinical Pearls."

Iyengar, B. K. S. Light on Pranayama.

Langer, Stephen, and James F. Scheer. Solved: The Riddle of Illness.

Maffetone, Phil. In Fitness and in Health.

Mandell, Marshall, and Theron G. Randolph. Dr. Mandell's Five-Day Allergy Relief System. New York: Harper & Row, 1988.

Philpott, William, and Dwight Kalita. Brain Allergies.: The Psycho-Nutrient Connection. New Canann, Conn.: Keats Publishing.

Randolph, Theron G., and Ralph W. Moss. An Alternative Approach to Allergies. New York: Harper & Row, 1980.

Steinman, David. Diet for a Poisoned Planet: How to Choose Safe Food for You and Your Family. New York: Crown Publishers, 1990.

Winter, Ruth. A Consumer's Dictionary of Food Additives. Rev. Ed. New York: Crown Publishers, 1984.

Wright, Jonathan. Dr. Wright's Guide to Healing With Nutrition.

PLEASE
USE
THE ORDER FORM
ON THE OTHER SIDE
OF THIS PAGE
TO EXPAND
YOUR WELL BEING
AND
GENERAL HEALTH

189

After reading this book, by now you can see the value of this information for making you feel wonderful. You can order more books for friends or, when you decide that you would like more resources by which you can ensure your good health, order a copy of the 30 Days to Total Energy tape set, using the form below or call us at 800-672-2250. You can fax us at 312-525-0050 or mail your order to: Arbor Vitae Communications, 124 N. York Rd. #230, Elmhurst, IL 60126.

Everything You Always Wanted to Know About Energy, But Were Too Tired to Ask	$14.95 + $2 S&H
Five or more copies	$9.95 + $2 S&H ea.
Thirty Days to Total Energy Tape Set	$69.95 + $3 S&H
Five or more sets	$49.95 + $3 S&H ea.

Six audio tapes containing NLP, hypnosis, meditation techniques and health information. The set includes a workbook that has nutritional information, recipes, menu plans and information about NLP and how to use the tapes for a complete and effective program to give you energy.

Tape 1 Side A: Introduction to the 30-day program. The triad of health.
Tape 1 Side B: Eliminating unwanted old habits. Developing desired new habits.

Tape 2 Side A: How to change your state of mind. Be in control of your emotions.
Tape 2 Side B: How to change your state of mind. Exercises to create energy, enthusiasm, confidence or any other desired emotion in an instant.

Tape 3 Side A: Physiology of sleep.
Tape 3 Side B: How to get to sleep and sleep well throughout the night.

Tape 4 Side A: Physiology of stress.
Tape 4 Side B: How to relax, eliminate stress and create healing.

Tape 5 Side A: Psychoneuroimmunology—healing and your mind.
Tape 5 Side B: Deep relaxation and healing.

Tape 6 Side A: Goal and direction setting. Getting what you want out of life.
Tape 6 Side B: Timeline.

Also by Dr. Varnas: FIFTY WAYS TO LOSE YOUR BLUBBER $9.95 + $2 S&H

Fill in number of copies desired:
_____ Tape Sets _____ *Everything You Always Wanted to Know About Energy*
_____ *Fifty Ways to Lose Your Blubber*

Total Amount $_____
Payment Method: O Check (enclosed) O MC O Visa O Disc O AX

_____
Account number   Expiration Date

_____
Signature

_____
Name

_____
Address   Apt

_____
City   State   Zip

190